Cancer Treatment and Research

Volume 173

Series editor

Steven T. Rosen, Duarte, CA, USA

More information about this series at http://www.springer.com/series/5808

William J. Gradishar

Editor

Optimizing Breast Cancer Management

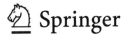 Springer

Editor
William J. Gradishar
Robert H. Lurie Comprehensive Cancer
    Center
Northwestern University Feinberg School
    of Medicine
Chicago, IL
USA

ISSN 0927-3042   ISSN 2509-8497   (electronic)
Cancer Treatment and Research
ISBN 978-3-319-88901-6   ISBN 978-3-319-70197-4   (eBook)
https://doi.org/10.1007/978-3-319-70197-4

Printed on acid-free paper

This Springer imprint is published by Springer Nature
The registered company is Springer International Publishing AG
The registered company address is: Gewerbestrasse 11, 6330 Cham, Switzerland

Contents

Strategies to Maintain Fertility in Young Breast Cancer Patients

1

Elizabeth S. Constance, Molly B. Moravek and Jacqueline S. Jeruss

Contents

E. S. Constance · M. B. Moravek
Department of Obstetrics and Gynecology, University of Michigan Health Systems,
Ann Arbor, MI, USA

J. S. Jeruss (✉)
Department of Surgery, University of Michigan, Ann Arbor, MI, USA
e-mail: jjeruss@med.umich.edu

J. S. Jeruss
Division of Surgical Oncology, 3303 Cancer Center, 1500 East Medical Center Drive,
Ann Arbor, MI 48109, USA

© Springer International Publishing AG 2018
W. J. Gradishar (ed.), *Optimizing Breast Cancer Management*, Cancer Treatment
and Research 173, https://doi.org/10.1007/978-3-319-70197-4_1

Abstract

Breast cancer is the most frequently occurring cancer in women of reproductive age. Treatments for breast cancer may eliminate or diminish fertility, making discussions about fertility preservation essential prior to initiation of gonadotoxic therapies. Additionally, even in patients who do not require chemotherapy, the use of adjuvant endocrine therapy will often push patients out of the reproductive window before treatment is completed. The only established methods for fertility preservation are oocyte or embryo cryopreservation, but experimental methods, such as ovarian suppression with GnRH agonists and ovarian tissue cryopreservation, show great promise. Early referral to a fertility specialist for interested patients affords patients the most fertility preservation options, with only minimal delay to cancer treatment.

Keywords

Fertility preservation · Oncofertility · Reproduction

1.1   Background

With improvements in early detection and treatment, breast cancer is becoming an increasingly curable disease with breast cancer survivors accounting for the largest group of female cancer survivors in the USA [27]. The overall five-year survival rate for breast cancer is now estimated at 92% among women younger than 45 years at the time of diagnosis [20]. Additionally, breast cancer is the most frequently occurring cancer in women of reproductive age, with approximately 12,500 cases diagnosed in women under the age of 40 each year in the USA [1]. Given that many women diagnosed with breast cancer will become long-term survivors, survivorship and quality of life issues, including reproductive health, are becoming increasingly important [10, 13].

Standard breast cancer treatments, such as systemic chemotherapy and adjuvant antihormonal treatments, can have both direct and indirect effects on long-term reproductive health including age-related fertility decline secondary to delayed childbearing and chemotherapy-induced ovarian failure. Infertility resulting from cancer treatment may be associated with significant psychosocial distress and decreased quality of life, sometimes leading patients to choose less efficacious treatment in order to decrease infertility risk [17, 18]. Therefore, for women of reproductive age preparing to undergo breast cancer treatment, referral to a reproductive specialist for discussion of fertility risks and preservation options is recommended. In order to reduce or eliminate delays in cancer treatment associated with fertility preservation, early referral, preferably at the time of breast cancer diagnosis, is critical. Furthermore, there is no evidence that currently used fertility preservation options negatively impact recurrence or survival rates [17].

Several national organizations, including the American Society of Clinical Oncology (ASCO), the National Comprehensive Cancer Network (NCCN), and the American Society for Reproductive Medicine (ASRM), have published guidelines supporting the discussion of fertility preservation with women of reproductive age, newly diagnosed with cancer, prior to the initiation of cancer treatment. ASCO published practice guidelines in 2006, recommending that oncologists address the possibility of infertility with patients treated during their reproductive years, and also be prepared to discuss possible fertility preservation options or refer interested patients to a reproductive specialist [17]. These guidelines were further updated in 2013, reiterating that healthcare providers, including medical oncologists, radiation oncologists, and surgeons, should address the risks of infertility associated with cancer therapies as part of the informed consent process and refer patients who express interest, as well as those who are undecided about fertility preservation, to an appropriate reproductive specialist [19]. Referrals should also be made for adolescents and younger patients who will receive gonadotoxic therapies [22].

Despite national guidelines and increasing healthcare provider awareness of these recommendations, pre-treatment fertility preservation services remain underutilized. A questionnaire administered to 60 women between the ages of 20–45 years, newly diagnosed with breast cancer, revealed that 50% of women desired children in the future or were unsure if they wanted children; however, only 9% received information about fertility preservation [10]. Another study, looking specifically at patient-provider discussions about the impact of cancer treatment on fertility in 104 women between the ages of 18–52 years, revealed that one-third of women were dissatisfied with the quality and length of discussions regarding the impact of cancer treatment on reproductive health, and only 14% of these women were encouraged to speak to a fertility specialist [26].

It may be difficult for providers to discern the significance of fertility preservation for young patients. Many patients do not bring up the topic of future fertility for a variety of reasons, including feeling overwhelmed by their cancer diagnosis, being unaware that loss of fertility may occur, or concerns about a potential treatment delay resulting in poor outcomes [19]. Therefore, it is incumbent upon the healthcare provider to ask women of reproductive age about their desires regarding future fertility so that appropriate and timely referral can be made. Improved multi-disciplinary collaboration between oncologists and reproductive specialists and widespread availability of fertility preservation services are necessary to expand the reproductive options of patients facing fertility-threatening therapies [22].

Pregnancy after breast cancer treatment should be considered acceptably safe. To date, studies have not indicated differences in disease-free survival or cancer recurrence rates as a result of subsequent pregnancy among women with both hormone receptor-positive and receptor-negative breast cancers [2, 16, 19]. Aside from patients identified to have genetic syndromes, there is no evidence that a history of cancer, cancer therapy, or fertility interventions increases the risk of issues such as genetic abnormalities, birth defects, or malignant neoplasms in the children of cancer survivors [17]. Additional prospective information regarding the safety of pregnancy after a breast diagnosis will be obtained from the IBCSG POSITIVE trial, which is currently accruing patients with a history of hormone receptor-positive breast cancer attempting pregnancy after treatment with two years of antihormonal therapy [18].

1.2 Effects of Cancer Treatment on Fertility

1.2.1 Oocyte Development and Fertility

Female gametogenesis takes place exclusively during the fetal period, thus at birth women have a fixed number of oocytes that do not regenerate over time. The number of oocytes peaks around 24 weeks of gestation and then begins to decline, with approximately 500,000–2 million oocytes remaining at birth [9]. Until puberty, the ovaries remain relatively quiescent, after which time they fall under the control of the hypothalamic–pituitary–ovarian axis. Pulsatile release of gonadotropin-releasing hormone (GnRH) from the hypothalamus results in secretion of the gonadotropins, follicle-stimulating hormone (FSH) and luteinizing hormone (LH) from the anterior pituitary. The hormone-producing granulosa and theca cells of the ovarian follicle, in turn, respond to cyclic changes in FSH and LH, leading to oocyte maturation and ovulation as well as sex hormone production, which has systemic effects including maintenance of bone and cardiovascular health. As the female germ cell population is fixed at birth, any insult to ovarian hormone production or oocyte reserve can have long-lasting detrimental effects on both fertility and overall health.

Most studies examining resumption of fertility following gonadotoxic therapy have looked at amenorrhea as a surrogate marker for infertility. The standard definition of amenorrhea is the absence of menses for six months or longer when not pregnant or using hormonal contraceptives [12]. Although many women will become amenorrheic while undergoing treatment with chemotherapy, over 90% who resume menses after treatment will do so within the first 12 months post-therapy [28]. It is important to note, however, that ovarian reserve may be diminished leading to infertility or a shortened reproductive window despite resumption of regular menses. Therefore, women who desire pregnancy following completion of gonadotoxic therapy should be referred early to a reproductive specialist regardless of menstrual regularity.

Compared with BRCA mutation-negative patients, some studies have shown BRCA mutation-positive women have lower baseline ovarian reserve even prior to the initiation of chemotherapy, with the BRCA1 mutation having the highest association with diminished ovarian reserve [21]. BRCA1 plays a role in the maintenance of double-stranded DNA breaks and telomere length, both of which are linked with reproductive life span [6]. It is hypothesized that patients with

BRCA mutations have oocytes which may be more prone to DNA damage, clinically manifesting as diminished ovarian reserve [25]. This decrease in baseline ovarian reserve may also result in greater susceptibility to chemotherapy-induced infertility. Similarly, BRCA mutation-positive women may have a less favorable response to controlled ovarian stimulation for oocyte retrieval when compared with age-matched controls without the mutation [16].

1.2.2 Chemotherapy

The effect of chemotherapy on reproductive health depends on the drug, dose, dose intensity, method of administration, disease, age, and pre-treatment fertility of the patient [17]. Women with breast cancer who receive chemotherapy such as alkylating agents and those over 40 years old may be more likely to experience amenorrhea and early menopause [12].

The current standard of therapy for the treatment of breast cancer is a multi-drug regimen consisting of adriamycin, cyclophosphamide, and a taxane. Among chemotherapy agents used to treat breast cancers, the greatest risk for impairment or destruction of ovarian reserve is associated with alkylating agents, including cyclophosphamide. Women who receive cyclophosphamide are four times more likely to experience ovarian failure than women who do not receive this agent [11]. The higher the cumulative dose of cyclophosphamide received, the greater the observed incidence of diminished ovarian reserve, infertility, and premature menopause [11].

1.2.3 Endocrine Therapies

For women with estrogen receptor-positive breast cancer, the use of adjuvant endocrine therapy is typically recommended for 5–10 years after diagnosis, with pregnancy being contraindicated during treatment because of teratogenic effects of antihormonal drugs. Although standard endocrine therapy, such as tamoxifen, does not produce direct damage to the ovaries, the lengthy treatment period can further delay childbearing for women who may already have reduced fertility caused by previous gonadotoxic therapy. As a result, many women may be perimenopausal or even postmenopausal by the time they complete adjuvant endocrine therapy [20].

1.2.4 Bioimmune Therapy

Trastuzumab, a monoclonal antibody targeting the HER2 receptor, is standard therapy for women with HER2-positive breast cancer. Available data examining the effects of trastuzumab on chemotherapy-related amenorrhea indicate no significant additive impact following one year of therapy [28].

1.2.5 Radiation Therapy

Localized and whole breast radiation used for treatment of breast cancer has minimal impact on ovarian reserve and subsequent fertility compared to the effects of systemic chemotherapy, although internal scatter radiation can have an indirect effect on the ovaries [11]. The degree to which radiotherapy impacts ovarian tissue is related to the volume treated, total radiation dose, fractionation schedule, and age at time of treatment [29]. The effective sterilizing dose of fractionated radiotherapy to the ovary at which premature ovarian failure occurs decreases with increasing age and is 18.4 Gy at age 20 years and 14.3 Gy at age 30 years; however, ovarian reserve is negatively impacted at doses as low as 2 Gy [29]. Due to concerns for potential radiation scatter, even with localized treatment to the breast, both ovarian stimulation for oocyte retrieval and pregnancy should be avoided during radiation treatment.

1.3 Oocyte and Embryo Cryopreservation

Controlled ovarian stimulation (COS) with cryopreservation of either mature oocytes or embryos is considered established treatment for fertility preservation. Recent advancements in COS protocols have resulted in improved safety for women with hormone-responsive malignancies and decreased time from referral to completion of fertility preservation treatment. Additionally, oocyte cryopreservation and embryo cryopreservation remain the most successful strategies to result in subsequent pregnancy. Therefore, oocyte and embryo cryopreservation should be offered to patients desiring fertility preservation as long as the patient's medical condition does not preclude COS [22].

The decision to cryopreserve mature oocytes versus embryos should be made on a case-by-case basis, taking into account the patient's relationship status as well as social, legal, and ethical considerations. As of 2013, the American Society for Reproductive Medicine (ASRM) no longer considers oocyte cryopreservation to be experimental, noting fertilization, clinical pregnancy, and live birth rates similar to those obtained with embryos developed from freshly retrieved oocytes [7, 22]. Legal concerns regarding custody and use of cryopreserved embryos in the case of divorce or dissolution of the relationship may lead to increased utilization of oocyte cryopreservation.

The number of oocytes obtained in a COS cycle is dependent on multiple individual factors including age, baseline ovarian reserve, and environmental factors affecting oocyte quality. Prior findings suggest that baseline ovarian reserve, response to COS, and oocyte yield may be impaired in women with cancer even before exposure to gonadotoxic therapies [22]. A meta-analysis of 227 untreated cancer patients and 1258 controls from seven studies reported a lower number of retrieved and mature oocytes in patients undergoing fertility preservation related to a cancer diagnosis [8]. In addition, due to age-related decline in oocyte number and quality, fertility preservation is expected to have lower success rates after age 40, and many fertility centers will have age cutoffs above which COS will not be offered.

The estimated overall oocyte to child efficiency is 6.7%, based on oocyte cryopreservation cycles not associated with cancer-related fertility preservation. The age-specific efficiencies of warmed oocytes are 7.4% for women less than 30 years old, 7.0% for women 30–34 years old, 6.5% for women 35–37 years old, and 5.2% for women over 38 years [7]. Therefore, cryopreservation of 15–20 metaphase II (MII) oocytes for women less than 38 years of age is expected to elicit a 70–80% chance of at least one live birth [7].

Embryos can be cryopreserved immediately after fertilization at the 2 pronuclear (2PN) stage on day one of embryo development, or at the blastocyst stage on day five of embryo development, with clinical pregnancy and live birth rates similar to fresh embryo transfer. While cryopreservation of embryos at the 2PN stage will lead to a higher number of cryopreserved embryos and thus may have some psychosocial benefit to the patient, cryopreservation at the blastocyst stage lends a more realistic picture of the chances of future pregnancy. Cryopreservation at the blastocyst phase also allows for embryo biopsy for preimplantation genetic screening for aneuploidy or preimplantation genetic diagnosis of hereditary genetic mutations such as BRCA mutations, prior to embryo cryopreservation.

1.3.1 Overview of Controlled Ovarian Stimulation

A controlled ovarian stimulation cycle takes approximately 2 weeks from start of medications to oocyte retrieval with a mean of 11.5 days and range of 9–20 days [25]. COS is achieved by daily subcutaneous injections of the gonadotropin hormones FSH and LH. Follicle size and estradiol levels are monitored by serial ultrasounds and/or serum hormone assays every 1–2 days while taking injectable gonadotropins. A gonadotropin-releasing hormone (GnRH) antagonist or agonist is also administered to prevent premature oocyte ovulation. Once an appropriate number of mature follicles are observed by ultrasound, initiation of the ovulation cascade is induced using either human chorionic gonadotropin (HCG) or GnRH agonist. Approximately 36 h after HCG or GnRH agonist administration, oocyte retrieval is performed via transvaginal ultrasound-guided needle aspiration of the ovarian follicles. Mature oocytes can be cryopreserved at the MII stage at that time or fertilized with either partner or donor sperm to create embryos that are then subsequently cryopreserved.

Risks associated with ovarian stimulation include development of ovarian hyperstimulation syndrome (OHSS), potential delay in initiation of cancer therapy, and risk of thromboembolic phenomena [22]. Modified COS protocols have subsequently been developed to address and minimize these risks.

1.3.2 Random-Start Protocols

Although COS protocols have traditionally initiated ovarian stimulation medications in the early follicular phase of the menstrual cycle, ovarian stimulation may begin at any point in the menstrual cycle without compromising oocyte quality or yield [5, 14]. These so-called random-start protocols allow increased access to fertility preservation treatment with minimal delays to the initiation cancer therapy.

Women with breast cancer may have an interval of 4–6 weeks between surgery and the initiation of adjuvant chemotherapy, with studies showing no effect on outcomes for patients with early-stage breast cancer if chemotherapy is initiated within 12 weeks after surgery [27]. This time frame will be sufficient in most cases to undergo COS for fertility preservation without causing a delay in care. However, for women requiring neoadjuvant chemotherapy, this timeline is much shorter. One study of fertility preservation in women with breast cancer showed that women who underwent neoadjuvant chemotherapy had only an average of 14 days between fertility preservation referral and initiation of chemotherapy when compared to 55 days for women who had surgery first. This time difference led to lower rates of utilization among women requiring neoadjuvant chemotherapy. In addition, this study found that the average time from cancer diagnosis to fertility preservation consult was 18 days, indicating that earlier referral at the time of diagnosis would allow for sufficient time to complete COS and oocyte retrieval without delaying the start of neoadjuvant chemotherapy [15]. Studies comparing random-start protocols with traditional early follicular phase protocols have shown similar efficacy [5, 14].

When appropriate, back-to-back ovarian stimulation and retrieval cycles may be completed in order to cryopreserve as many oocytes or embryos as possible, thus maximizing the probability of a live birth in the future without unduly delaying time-sensitive cancer therapy [27]. A non-randomized study of women undergoing fertility preservation prior to breast cancer treatment found that the timing of referral for fertility preservation directly correlated with the number of oocyte retrieval cycles completed. This study found that patients completing two oocyte retrieval cycles were more likely to be referred prior to breast cancer surgery when compared to patients completing only one cycle. There was no difference in the time interval from initial diagnosis to initiation of chemotherapy between the two groups, and no difference in incidence of breast cancer recurrence was observed between the two groups after 67 months of follow-up [27].

1.3.3 Use of Adjunct Aromatase Inhibitor

One of the primary concerns for both patients and oncologists regarding fertility preservation is the risk of advancing hormone-responsive cancers through the process of ovarian stimulation. Therefore, ovarian stimulation protocols have been developed which combine use of gonadotropins with an aromatase inhibitor in order to suppress estradiol levels associated with ovarian hyperstimulation and maintain estradiol near physiologic levels. The most commonly used aromatase inhibitor for COS in breast cancer patients is letrozole, a potent and highly selective third-generation aromatase inhibitor. Letrozole is preferred, secondary to the association with higher numbers of oocytes obtained and fertilized without increased adverse events [3, 25].

These protocols are well tolerated and yield similar numbers of oocytes and embryos compared to standard protocols, while minimizing the risk of high estrogen exposure in women with hormone-sensitive malignancies [5]. To date, data show no increased risk of recurrence and no difference in relapse-free survival when letrozole was added to an FSH-based COS regimen [4, 15]. Therefore, COS with concomitant letrozole administration is considered both reasonable and effective for breast cancer patients pursuing fertility preservation.

1.3.4 Ovarian Hyperstimulation Syndrome

Ovarian hyperstimulation syndrome (OHSS) is a risk associated with all COS cycles. This syndrome is caused by VEGF-mediated vascular hyper-permeability leading to intravascular depletion and third spacing of fluids resulting from multiple luteinized follicles within the ovary. Because symptoms of OHSS including dehydration, nausea, vomiting, and pulmonary edema can interfere with and delay initiation of chemotherapy, minimizing the development and progression of OHSS is an important factor in fertility preservation before cancer treatment. Because OHSS is exacerbated by high HCG levels, use of a GnRH agonist rather than HCG to trigger the ovulation cascade has been shown to reduce estrogen exposure and improve cycle outcomes by increasing the yield of mature oocytes and embryos as well as decreasing the incidence of OHSS [14].

1.4 Ovarian Suppression

Ovarian suppression with a GnRH agonist during chemotherapy is still considered investigational at this time. Use of GnRH agonists causes down-regulation of the GnRH neurons following an initial increase in activity, or "flare." This down-regulation inhibits the pulsatile release of gonadotropins from the anterior pituitary leading to a menopause-like cessation of ovarian follicle growth and development. It is theorized that this inhibition of follicle growth makes the developing oocytes and hormone-producing cells of the ovary less transcriptionally active and therefore less sensitive to the gonadotoxic effects of chemotherapy, potentially preserving post-treatment fertility and endogenous hormone production [14]. In addition to the potential fertility and hormonal benefits, GnRH agonists may have other medical benefits including menstrual suppression leading to a reduction in vaginal bleeding when patients have low platelet counts as a result of chemotherapy [19].

The Prevention of Early Menopause Study (POEMS) evaluated premenopausal women age 25–49 years with hormone receptor-negative breast cancer and found that 33% of patients who underwent chemotherapy without ovarian suppression subsequently met the criteria for ovarian dysfunction, defined as amenorrhea in the preceding 6 months and FSH levels in the postmenopausal range, whereas only 14% of women who underwent chemotherapy with adjunct ovarian suppression met these criteria at the two-year end point [10]. This study also found that disease-free survival was significantly better in the experimental arm in this patient population [16].

The PROMISE trial (Prevention of Menopause Induced by Chemotherapy: A Study in Early Breast Cancer Patients) further evaluated women with both hormone receptor-negative and receptor-positive breast cancers, with 80% of trial participants having hormone receptor-positive disease [28]. This study found a doubling in the number of pregnancies and trend toward increased probability of menstrual resumption in women undergoing chemotherapy with ovarian suppression. Importantly, the study did not find differences in disease-free survival between the treatment arms, including a subgroup analysis of the hormone receptor-positive cohort [16]. To date, a total of six randomized controlled trials and eight subsequent meta-analyses of these data have been performed. The majority of these studies show potential efficacy of this therapy; however, further study and longer follow-up are needed before this treatment can be considered standard therapy.

1.5 Ovarian Tissue Cryopreservation

Ovarian tissue cryopreservation is an investigational option for fertility preservation, currently only available under institutional review board-approved protocols at select hospitals across the country. In this technique, part or all of an ovary is surgically removed prior to the initiation of chemotherapy, and ovarian cortical strips are then cryopreserved. These cryopreserved ovarian strips can later be thawed and autotransplanted either orthotopically, onto the patient's remaining ovary, or heterotopically in the forearm, abdominal wall, or chest wall. Ovarian tissue cryopreservation theoretically represents an efficient method of preserving thousands of ovarian follicles at one time [22]. Transplanted ovarian tissue allows for resumption of both endogenous hormone production and potential fertility.

This technique has been proposed principally for prepubertal girls and for those women who cannot delay cancer treatment in order to undergo ovarian stimulation and oocyte retrieval [22, 23]. In postmenarchal women, resumption of normal ovulatory menstrual cycles has been reported to occur within 4–9 months after transplantation which is consistent with the time necessary to initiation follicle growth and maturation [23]. Studies have shown variability in graft survival and ovarian function, from several months to years depending on the amount of tissue transplanted, as well as the age and ovarian reserve of the woman when the ovarian tissue was excised, with the longest documented graft survival lasting 7 years [23]. To date, live births have been reported with orthotopic transplantation only.

Risks associated with ovarian tissue transplantation include the surgical and anesthetic risk involved with obtaining tissue and subsequent re-implantations. Ovarian tissue cryopreservation is not currently recommended for BRCA mutation carriers, secondary to the risk of associated ovarian cancers and concern regarding the potential risk of reseeding occult malignant cells after tissue transplantation [14].

Ovarian tissue cryopreservation is a promising and emerging field in fertility preservation and may be the only option for women with aggressive disease who cannot delay treatment in order to undergo ovarian stimulation and oocyte retrieval. Women should be counseled regarding the investigational nature of this procedure and be referred in an expedited fashion to an appropriate facility if interested in pursuing this option.

1.6 In Vitro Oocyte Maturation

Development of fertility preservation technologies that both reduce patient risk and minimize delay in treatment is an important and rapidly growing field within reproductive medicine. Basic laboratory research is currently being conducted to develop methods of isolating and maturing oocytes and follicles at all stages of development from both fresh and previously cryopreserved ovarian tissues [22].

In vitro oocyte maturation (IVM) involves maturation of immature oocytes in the laboratory for cryopreservation of mature oocytes or fertilization for embryo cryopreservation. Advantages of this approach over conventional ovary stimulation and oocyte retrieval include increased flexibility, avoidance of large doses of gonadotropins, decreased cost associated with stimulation medications, and minimal exposure to elevated estradiol levels [25]. The first successful pregnancy achieved via this method was reported in 2014; however, this technique is still considered investigational because long-term safety and efficacy are unknown [22, 24]. No live births have been reported from intraoperative recovery of immature oocytes at the time of harvesting ovarian tissue for cryopreservation followed by in vitro maturation, although this is an area of ongoing research interest [23]. Cryopreservation of immature oocytes for later IVM has also been proposed but is still considered experimental [14]. The ability to grow and mature oocytes in vitro would allow for future fertility while mitigating the risks associated with autotransplantation of previously cryopreserved ovarian tissue including concerns regarding seeding of occult malignant cells and need for multiple surgeries due to shortened graft life.

1.7 Conclusion

As early detection and treatment of breast cancer continue to improve, increasing numbers of women are becoming long-term survivors highlighting concerns regarding long-term health and quality of life after cancer treatment. For women of reproductive age, one of the greatest issues regarding long-term survival is the ability to have children when desired. It is imperative for oncologists to discuss the impact of cancer treatments on future fertility with women of reproductive age as part of the informed consent process for treatment. Early referral to a reproductive specialist at the time of a new cancer diagnosis is essential to allow women to be informed about the full range of fertility preservation options. Several fertility preservation options exist, allowing for patients to make personalized decisions regarding future family building without delaying initiation of life-saving cancer therapies or impacting long-term survival.

References

1. American Cancer Society (2015) Breast cancer facts & figures 2015-2016. American Cancer Society, Inc., Atlanta
2. Azim HA Jr, Kroman N, Paesmans M, Gelber S, Rotmensz N, Ameye L, De Mattos-Arruda L, Pistilli B, Pinto A, Jensen MB, Cordoba O, de Azambuja E, Goldhirsch A, Piccart MJ, Peccatori FA (2013) Prognostic impact of pregnancy after breast cancer according to estrogen receptor status: a multicenter retrospective study. J Clin Oncol 31(1):73–79
3. Bedoschi G, Oktay K (2013) Current approach to fertility preservation by embryo cryopreservation. Fertil Steril 99(6):1496–1502
4. Boukaidi SA, Cooley A, Hardy A, Matthews L, Zelivianski S, Jeruss JS (2012) Impact of infertility regimens on breast cancer cells: follicle-stimulating hormone and luteinizing hormone lack a direct effect on breast cell proliferation in vitro. Fertil Steril 97(2):440–444
5. Cakmak H, Rosen MP (2015) Random-start ovarian stimulation in patients with cancer. Curr Opin Obstet Gynecol 27(3):215–221
6. Diaz de la Noval B (2016) Potential implications on female fertility and reproductive lifespan in BRCA germline mutation women. Arch Gynecol Obstet 294(5):1099–1103
7. Doyle JO, Richter KS, Lim J, Stillman RJ, Graham JR, Tucker MJ (2016) Successful elective and medically indicated oocyte vitrification and warming for autologous in vitro fertilization, with predicted birth probabilities for fertility preservation according to number of cryopreserved oocytes and age at retrieval. Fertil Steril 105(2):459–466 e452
8. Friedler S, Koc O, Gidoni Y, Raziel A, Ron-El R (2012) Ovarian response to stimulation for fertility preservation in women with malignant disease: a systematic review and meta-analysis. Fertil Steril 97(1):125–133
9. Fritz M, Speroff L (2011) Clinical gynecologic endocrinology and infertility, 8th edn. Lippincott Williams & Wilkins, Philadelphia
10. Goldfarb SB, Kamer SA, Oppong BA, Eaton A, Patil S, Junqueira MJ, Olcese C, Kelvin JF, Gemignani ML (2016) Fertility preservation for the young breast cancer patient. Ann Surg Oncol 23(5):1530–1536
11. Goncalves V, Quinn GP (2016) Review of fertility preservation issues for young women with breast cancer. Hum Fertil (Camb) 1–14
12. Jacobson MH, Mertens AC, Spencer JB, Manatunga AK, Howards PP (2016) Menses resumption after cancer treatment-induced amenorrhea occurs early or not at all. Fertil Steril 105(3):765–772 e764

13. Jeruss JS, Woodruff TK (2009) Preservation of fertility in patients with cancer. N Engl J Med 360(9):902–911. PMID: 19246362
14. Kasum M, von Wolff M, Franulic D, Cehic E, Klepac-Pulanic T, Oreskovic S, Juras J (2015) Fertility preservation options in breast cancer patients. Gynecol Endocrinol 31(11):846–851
15. Kim J, Oktay K, Gracia C, Lee S, Morse C, Mersereau JE (2012) Which patients pursue fertility preservation treatments? A multicenter analysis of the predictors of fertility preservation in women with breast cancer. Fertil Steril 97(3):671–676
16. Lambertini M, Ginsburg ES, Partridge AH (2015) Update on fertility preservation in young women undergoing breast cancer and ovarian cancer therapy. Curr Opin Obstet Gynecol 27 (1):98–107
17. Lee SJ, Schover LR, Partridge AH, Patrizio A, Wallace LN, Hagerty LV, Beck LN, Brennan LV, Oktay K, American Society of Clinical (2006) American Society of Clinical Oncology recommendations on fertility preservation in cancer patients. J Clin Oncol 24 (18):2917–2931
18. Llarena NC, Estevez SL, Tucker SL, Jeruss JS (2015) Impact of fertility concerns on tamoxifen initiation and persistence. JNCI J Natl Cancer Inst 107(10). PMID: 26307641
19. Loren AW, Mangu PB, Beck LN, Brennan L, Magdalinski AJ, Partridge AH, Quinn G, Wallace WH, Oktay K, American Society of Clinical (2013) Fertility preservation for patients with cancer: American Society of Clinical Oncology clinical practice guideline update. J Clin Oncol 31(19):2500–2510
20. McCray DK, Simpson AB, Flyckt R, Liu Y, O'Rourke C, Crowe JP, Grobmyer SR, Moore HC, Valente SA (2016) Fertility in women of reproductive age after breast cancer treatment: practice patterns and outcomes. Ann Surg Oncol 23(10):3175–3181
21. Oktay K, Kim JY, Barad D, Babayev SN (2009) Association of BRCA1 mutations with occult primary ovarian insufficiency: a possible explanation for the link between infertility and breast/ovarian cancer risks. J Clin Oncol 28(2):240–244
22. Practice Committee of American Society for Reproductive (2013) Fertility preservation in patients undergoing gonadotoxic therapy or gonadectomy: a committee opinion. Fertil Steril 100(5):1214–1223
23. Practice Committee of American Society for Reproductive (2014) Ovarian tissue cryopreservation: a committee opinion. Fertil Steril 101(5):1237–1243
24. Prasath EB, Chan ML, Wong WH, Lim CJ, Tharmalingam MD, Hendricks M, Loh SF, Chia YN (2014) First pregnancy and live birth resulting from cryopreserved embryos obtained from in vitro matured oocytes after oophorectomy in an ovarian cancer patient. Hum Reprod 29(2):276–278
25. Reddy J, Oktay K (2012) Ovarian stimulation and fertility preservation with the use of aromatase inhibitors in women with breast cancer. Fertil Steril 98(6):1363–1369
26. Scanlon M, Blaes A, Geller M, Majhail NS, Lindgren B, Haddad T (2012) Patient satisfaction with physician discussions of treatment impact on fertility, menopause and sexual health among pre-menopausal women with cancer. J Cancer 3:217–225
27. Turan V, Bedoschi G, Moy F, Oktay K (2013) Safety and feasibility of performing two consecutive ovarian stimulation cycles with the use of letrozole-gonadotropin protocol for fertility preservation in breast cancer patients. Fertil Steril 100(6):1681–1685 e1681
28. Waks AG, Partridge AH (2016) Fertility preservation in patients with breast cancer: necessity, methods, and safety. JNCCN 14(3):355–363
29. Wallace WH, Thomson AB, Saran F, Kelsey TW (2005) Predicting age of ovarian failure after radiation to a field that includes the ovaries. Int J Radiat Oncol Biol Phys 62(3):738–744

Adjuvant Endocrine Therapy

2

Rena Shah and Ruth M. O'Regan

Contents

Abstract

The use of hormonal therapy in breast cancer has improved the overall outcome for patients with early-stage hormone receptor-positive disease. The choice of hormone therapy is related to multiple factors, including menopausal state, patient preference, and potential side effects. Molecular profiling has allowed therapy to be tailored for an individual patient to some extent. However, further molecular studies are needed to individualize the choice and length of adjuvant hormone therapy. Ongoing studies are evaluating the role of additional targeted

R. Shah · R. M. O'Regan (✉)
University of Wisconsin Carbone Cancer Center, Madison, USA
e-mail: roregan@medicine.wisc.edu

© Springer International Publishing AG 2018
W. J. Gradishar (ed.), *Optimizing Breast Cancer Management*, Cancer Treatment and Research 173, https://doi.org/10.1007/978-3-319-70197-4_2

therapies, such as CDK4/6 inhibitors, to further improve outcome for patients with early-stage hormone receptor-positive breast cancer.

Keywords

Breast cancer · Adjuvant · Endocrine therapy · Hormone therapy
Tamoxifen · Aromatase inhibitors · Molecular profiling

2.1   Introduction

Approximately two-thirds of breast cancers are hormone receptor (HR)-positive defined by their expression of estrogen and/or progesterone receptors. The use of endocrine therapy has been shown to significantly improve outcome in patients with all stages of HR-positive breast cancer. Adjuvant endocrine therapies decrease recurrence by approximately one-third in patients with early-stage HR-positive breast cancer. Tamoxifen is a selective estrogen receptor modulator (SERM) that prevents dimerization of the estrogen receptor (ER), thereby acting as an anti-estrogen on breast and other tissues. Aromatase inhibitors (AIs) block the peripheral conversion of androgens to estrogen in postmenopausal women and have shown modestly improved outcome compared to tamoxifen.

Despite the success of endocrine agents in preventing HR-positive breast cancer recurrence, a significant proportion of patients relapse, due in large part to endocrine resistance. Genomic profiling has demonstrated the existence of at least two subtypes of HR-positive breast cancer, referred to as luminal A and luminal B. Luminal A cancers are characterized by high expression of hormone receptors, low proliferation indices, and sensitivity to endocrine agents. In contrast, luminal B cancers express lower levels of ER, are often progesterone receptor (PR)-negative, have high proliferation and likely intrinsic resistance to endocrine therapy. A better understanding of the biology of an individual patient's HR-positive breast cancer is becoming possible with available genomic assays and will likely lead to novel therapeutic approaches for patients with endocrine-resistant cancers, thereby improving outcome.

2.2   Biomarkers in HR-Positive Breast Cancer

2.2.1   Hormone Receptors

Breast cancers are defined by their expression of HR, namely, ER and PR, and HER2. Current guidelines classify breast cancers as HR-positive if they express $\geq 1\%$ of either ER or PR by immunohistochemisty [2]. It is clear that breast cancers that express $\leq 10\%$ of HR benefit less from endocrine therapy (ASCO-CAP guidelines 2010). The majority of breast cancers in both pre- and postmenopausal women are HR-positive. Although the recurrence rate is lower for HR-positive, compared to HR-negative breast cancers, during 5 years following diagnosis, these cancers continue to recur many years following diagnosis, reflecting a tumor dormancy the biology of which is, to date, not well understood.

The presence of HR is associated with benefit from endocrine agents, which has improved outcomes for patients with all stages of HR-positive breast cancers. However, from genomic analyses, it is apparent that there are at least two subtypes of HR-positive breast cancer that have different prognoses and likely require tailored therapeutic approaches [28].

2.2.2 Molecular Profiling

As noted above, there are at least two distinct HR-positive breast cancer subtypes—luminal A and luminal B. Luminal A cancers, characterized by high HR expression and low proliferation, appear to obtain minimal benefit from adjuvant chemotherapy, but likely benefit significantly from endocrine therapy, whereas luminal B cancers, with lower HR expression and high proliferation, are more likely to be resistant to endocrine therapy, which contributes to their inferior outcome compared to luminal A cancers [28]. A number of genomic assays have been developed to determine prognosis and help tailor adjuvant therapy for patients with early-stage HR-positive breast cancer.

2.2.2.1 Molecular Profiling at Initial Diagnosis

The 21-gene recurrence score (RS) (Oncotype DX) comprises 16 cancer genes and 5 reference genes and has been demonstrated to be prognostic and predictive of chemotherapy benefit in patients with node-negative HR-positive breast cancer [23, 24] (Table 2.1). Initial data, utilizing specimens from the NSABP B-14 trial which evaluated the use of adjuvant tamoxifen, showed that 21-gene RS is prognostic for patients with node-negative HR-positive breast cancer, treated with 5 years of endocrine therapy [11, 23]. Further, this assay was found to be predictive of benefit of chemotherapy in patients with node-negative HR-positive breast cancers, using specimens from the NSABP B-20 trial [24]. Prospective analysis of the 21-gene RS is being evaluated in the TAILORx trial, in which patients are treated based on the RS. Initial data from this trial [29] demonstrate a favorable prognosis for patients with cancers with RS $\leq$ 10 who received endocrine therapy alone. The 21-gene RS has additionally been shown to be prognostic and predictive of chemotherapy benefit in patients with node-positive HR-positive breast cancer, though this study included a relatively small number of patients. Prospective evaluation of the 21-gene RS is ongoing in the SWOG 1007 trial. Unpublished data from the NSABP B-14 trial suggest that the 21-gene RS is predictive of benefit from endocrine therapy, with patients with cancers with high RS obtaining minimal benefit from the use of tamoxifen [23].

The 70-gene signature (MammaPrint) has been demonstrated to be prognostic in patients with early-stage breast cancer with up to three involved nodes (Table 2.1).

Table 2.1 Selected completed or ongoing analyses evaluating molecular profiling in early-stage breast cancer

Molecular profile	Trial for validation	Patient population	Gene	Determination	N	Comments
21-gene recurrence score (Oncotype DX)	NSABP-B14 (prospective-retrospective) [23]	Women with stage I/II, HR +, lymph node-negative, invasive carcinoma, treated with tamoxifen or placebo	21-gene, DNA microarray	Likelihood of distant recurrence at 10 years from diagnosis	668	Approved by ASCO (2007), NCCN (2011), NICE (2013)
	NSABP-B20 (prospective-retrospective) [24]	Women with stage I/II, HR +, lymph node-negative, invasive carcinoma, treated with tamoxifen or chemotherapy with tamoxifen		Likelihood of distant recurrence at 10 years from diagnosis	651	ASCO (2007), NCCN (2011), NICE (2013)
	TAILORx (prospective)	Women with stage I/II, HR +, lymph node-negative, invasive carcinoma, tumor size <5.0 cm		Outcome for patients with low-risk cancers treated with endocrine therapy; cutoff of chemotherapy benefit	10,253	Ongoing, favorable five-year outcome in low-risk group [29]
	SWOG 8614 (prospective-retrospective) [1]	HR+, node-positive breast cancer treated with tamoxifen or chemotherapy followed by tamoxifen		Disease-free survival	367	No chemotherapy benefit in low-risk group
	SWOG 1007	HR+, N1 breast cancer with recurrence score ≤25 randomized to chemotherapy followed by endocrine therapy or endocrine therapy alone		Disease-free survival	5600	Completed accrual

(continued)

Table 2.1 (continued)

Molecular profile	Trial for validation	Patient population	Gene	Determination	N	Comments
70-gene signature (MammaPrint)	MINDACT trial (phase III, prospective)	Women with stage I/II, 0–3 positive lymph nodes, invasive carcinoma, tumor size <5.0 cm	70-gene, formalin fixed or fresh tissue DNA microarray analysis	Determine high versus low risk for recurrence – high risk, recommend chemotherapy – low risk, recommend hormonal therapy alone	6693	FDA approved (2007) Low-risk group favorable outcome without chemotherapy
EndoPredict (EPclin)	Buus, JNCI [4]; compared to OncoType DX Subset of transATAC	ER-positive, HER2 negative, treated with adjuvant endocrine therapy only	11-gene, formalin fixed or fresh tissue qRT-PCR assay with nodal size and tumor size	Distant recurrence, disease relapse-free survival over 10 years	964	
BCI	Subset of transATAC; MA 17	HR-positive, lymph node-negative, in ATAC trial		Distant recurrence, disease relapse-free survival over 10 years	665	BCI prognostic for late recurrence; H/I ratio predictive of extended AI
IHC4	Subset of transATAC;	HR-positive, lymph node-negative, in ATAC trial	IHC for ER, PR, HER2, Ki67	Distant recurrence, disease relapse-free survival over 10 years	786	
PAM50	MA.12 [6]	Any HR status after adjuvant chemotherapy	50-gene, qRT-PCR	Prognostic for disease-free survival and overall survival and predicting benefit with tamoxifen therapy	672	

The MINDACT trial [5] estimated risk of recurrence using classical clinical criteria along with the 70-gene signature. Patients who were deemed low risk by both methods did not receive chemotherapy and received endocrine therapy if their cancers were HR-positive; patients who were deemed high risk by both methods received chemotherapy; patients with discordant risk using the two methods were randomized to receive chemotherapy or not. Similar to the TAILORx study, the MINDACT trial identified a group of patients with low-risk cancers who had an excellent prognosis without chemotherapy. Interestingly, there was no benefit for adjuvant chemotherapy in either of the discordant groups.

A number of other molecular assays, including the intrinsic gene analysis (PAM50) and EndoPredict (Table 2.1), are also available for risk analysis in patients with early-stage HR-positive breast cancer. Overall, the use of these molecular profiles has improved the understanding of the biology of these cancers, allowing tailoring of adjuvant therapies and importantly avoiding the use of chemotherapy in patients who are unlikely to benefit.

2.2.2.2 Molecular Profiling to Determine Benefit of Extended Adjuvant Endocrine Therapy

The Breast Cancer Index (BCI) comprises HOXB13:IL17BR (H/I) ratio along with molecular grade index and has been shown to be prognostic of late (years 5–10) recurrences [27] (Table 2.1). The HOXB13 gene is part of the homeobox family, found on chromosome 17, and men who inherit a variant form of the gene have an increased risk of prostate cancer. HOXB13 expression was associated with a shorter relapse-free survival, whereas increased expression of IL17BR is associated with a longer relapse-free survival. BCI is comprised of seven genes, including H/I ratio and molecular grade index, to help patients better understand the potential benefits of an additional five years of endocrine therapy, based on MA.14 data, which evaluated anti-estrogen therapy with or without octreotide therapy in post-menopausal women [27] (Table 2.2). The H/I ratio was evaluated in the MA.17 trial (Table 2.3) to predict the likelihood of late recurrences (years 5 through 10 from diagnosis) as well as the benefit from extended letrozole therapy. A number of other molecular assays have also been evaluated in predicting recurrence beyond 5 years. However, BCI is the only assay that has been evaluated in patients who have received extended adjuvant therapy though this involved a relatively small subset of the MA.17 trial. Further validation of this assay is ongoing.

2.3 Adjuvant Endocrine Therapy

2.3.1 Menopausal Status

In premenopausal women, estrogen production is primarily provided by the ovaries, whereas, in postmenopausal women, the primary source of estradiol is the conversion via the aromatase enzyme in adrenal glands, along with other tissues. As

Table 2.2 Postmenopausal adjuvant hormonal therapy

Trial	Comparator	Study population	N	Level of evidence	Primary end point	Median follow-up	Outcome
ATAC [17]	Anastrozole versus tamoxifen for total 5 years	HR+, localized invasive carcinoma	6241	Phase III	DFS	68 months	Anastrozole superior to tamoxifen but no difference in survival
MA.27 [14]	Anastrozole versus exemestane for total 5 years	HR+, localized invasive carcinoma	7576	Phase III	DFS	4.1 years	Anastrozole equivalent to exemestane
BIG 1–98 [3]	Letrozole versus tamoxifen for total 5 years	HR+, localized invasive carcinoma	8010	Phase III	DFS	25.8 months	Letrozole superior to tamoxifen
ARNO 95 [18]	Tamoxifen for 5 years versus tamoxifen for 2 years to anastrozole for total 5 years	HR+, localized invasive carcinoma	1040	Phase III	Overall survival	30.1 months	Tamoxifen followed by anastrozole improved overall survival compared to continued tamoxifen
Intergroup Exemestane study [7]	Tamoxifen for 5 years versus tamoxifen for 2–3 years to exemestane for total 5 years	HR+, localized invasive carcinoma	4742	Phase III	DFS	30.6 months	Tamoxifen followed by exemestane improved overall survival compared to continued tamoxifen

Table 2.3 Extended adjuvant hormonal therapy

Trial	Design	Prior therapy	N	Primary end point	Results
ATLAS [8]	Tamoxifen for 10 years versus 5 years	HR+, localized invasive carcinoma	12,894	Overall survival	Decreased recurrence and improved mortality after 10 years
aTTom [16]	Tamoxifen for 5 years versus control	Tamoxifen for 5 years, HR+, localized invasive carcinoma	6953	DFS	Decreased recurrence after 10 years
MA.17 [13]	Letrozole versus placebo for total 5 years	After 5 years of tamoxifen, HR+	5187	DFS	Improved DFS overall and improved distant DFS and survival in node-positive disease
MA.17R [14]	Letrozole for 5 years versus placebo	Tamoxifen for 3–5 years followed by AI for 5 years	1918	DFS	Positive for DFS but did not include deaths from other causes, benefit primarily in contralateral breast cancer occurrence
NSABP B-42 [19, 20]	Letrozole for 5 years versus placebo	AI for 5 years or Tamoxifen followed by AI for total 5 years	3923	Disease-free survival	No statistically significant benefit in primary end point or overall survival, letrozole arm showed benefit in breast-cancer-free interval and in distant recurrence
SOLE (NCT00553410)	Continuous versus intermittent letrozole for 5 years	Endocrine therapy for 5 years	4800	Disease-free survival	Ongoing

defined by the NCCN guidelines, menopause is when there is a lack of estrogen synthesis from the ovaries. Criteria for postmenopausal state are met in the setting of prior bilateral oophorectomies, age greater than or equal to 60, or less than 60 with no menses for at least 12 months without the use of chemotherapy, ovarian suppression, or anti-estrogen therapy, with FSH and estradiol is in the post-menopausal range. Of note, if a patient is on LHRH agonist or antagonist, menopausal status cannot be determined. If a woman's menopausal status cannot be determined, they should be treated as premenopausal with tamoxifen, since AIs are largely ineffective in these women.

2.3.2 Endocrine Therapy Classification

2.3.2.1 Selective Estrogen Receptor Modulators

Tamoxifen is a selective estrogen receptor modulator (SERM) that competitively antagonizes the estrogen receptor by blocking its dimerization, thereby inhibiting the growth of the HR-positive breast cancer cells. It is most commonly considered in the premenopausal women but is additionally used in postmenopausal women who cannot tolerate an aromatase inhibitor. Use of adjuvant tamoxifen for up to 5 years was shown to reduce breast cancer death rate by 31% versus placebo in the EBCTCG meta-analysis [10]. Major side effects of tamoxifen include increased risk of thromboembolic disease, cerebrovascular accidents, and uterine cancer, predominantly in postmenopausal women. More commonly, tamoxifen causes side effects consistent with menopause including hot flashes, sexual dysfunction, and vaginal discharge. Resistance to tamoxifen is multifactorial, including, loss of ER-expression, up-regulation of growth factors, and altered drug metabolization via the CYP2D6 enzyme. Concomitant use of CYP2D6 inhibitors has been shown to decrease the efficacy of tamoxifen in several, but not all studies [25]. In women unable to tolerate tamoxifen, another SERM, toremifene, which is a chlorinated derivative of tamoxifen, has been shown to have equal efficacy and similar toxicity, though it is not approved in the USA as an adjuvant therapy.

While on tamoxifen therapy, it is recommended for women to use contraception as treatment can induce ovulation. In addition, waiting for 2–3 months from therapy cessation for conception is recommended. However, if a patient becomes pregnant while on therapy, tamoxifen should be discontinued as it associated with congenital anomalies.

2.3.2.2 Aromatase Inhibitors

AIs block the peripheral conversion of androgens to estrogen. Compared to tamoxifen, use of AIs has been demonstrated to modestly improve outcomes in HR-positive disease in the postmenopausal setting, specifically in modestly improving the rate of relapse. As postmenopausal women have non-functioning ovaries, AIs are most effective in this setting and not recommended in premenopausal women, including in those with chemotherapy-induced amenorrhea. All of the currently utilized AIs, letrozole, anastrozole, exemestane, are specific for the aromatase enzyme and have improved toxicity profiles, compared to previous AIs. A number of pivotal studies (Table 2.2) demonstrated superiority of AIs compared to tamoxifen. The ATAC (Arimidex, Tamoxifen alone, or Combination) trial compared 5 years of anastrozole to 5 years of tamoxifen or to the combination of both agents and showed an improved disease-free survival for anastrozole over tamoxifen [17]. The BIG 1-98 trial [3] demonstrated improved outcome with letrozole compared to tamoxifen, both given for 5 years. This trial additionally demonstrated that tamoxifen for 2 years followed by letrozole for 3 years, or letrozole for 2 years followed by tamoxifen for 3 years was equivalent to letrozole for 5 years, with all three treatment arms being superior to tamoxifen for 5 years. Similarly, NSABP-B33 showed a four-year relapse-free survival advantage in the exemestane group compared to placebo [7]. Adverse effects from AIs include musculoskeletal side effects (AIMSS—aromatase inhibitor-associated musculoskeletal syndrome), osteoporosis, and possibly increased cardiovascular risks, along with sexual dysfunction, including dyspareunia, decreased vaginal lubrication, and decreased libido. AIMSS is typically managed with early exercises and NSAIDs.

2.3.2.3 Ovarian Suppression

Ovarian suppression or ablation inhibits estrogen production from the ovaries either permanently through oophorectomy or pelvic radiation or temporarily through gonadotropin-releasing hormone (GnRH) agonists. With permanent ovarian function cessation, patients are at an increased risk of cardiovascular disease and osteoporosis, along with the expected side effects of menopause. Two large randomized trials demonstrated improved outcome for a subset of premenopausal women with HR-positive early-stage breast cancer treated with the addition of ovarian suppression to endocrine therapy. In the SOFT (Suppression of Ovarian Function) trial, premenopausal women with HR-positive early-stage breast cancer were randomized to tamoxifen alone, tamoxifen with ovarian suppression, or exemestane with ovarian suppression. The TEXT (Tamoxifen and Exemestane) trial evaluated ovarian suppression with tamoxifen versus ovarian suppression with exemestane in premenopausal women with HR-positive early-stage breast cancer [22]. Combined analysis of the studies showed an improved five-year disease-free survival with ovarian suppression with exemestane over tamoxifen, which appeared, however, to be restricted to younger women and those who received chemotherapy. Ovarian suppression induces short-term side effects associated with menopause and the probability of long-term issues with bone loss and possible premature coronary artery disease. Therefore, a biomarker associated with benefit from this more toxic approach would be beneficial in selecting patients most likely to benefit.

2.3.3   Choice of Therapy Based on Menopausal Status

2.3.3.1   Premenopausal Women

Though tamoxifen remains a standard of care, results of the SOFT/TEXT trials support the addition of ovarian suppression with exemestane in patients considered at high risk of recurrence, which is supported by NCCN guidelines. While criteria for high-risk features are not entirely established, the following conditions are considered high risk: larger tumor size, high tumor grade, lymphovascular invasion, positive lymph nodes, recommendation for chemotherapy, and high risk of recurrence as determined by a genomic assay. Of note, NCCN considers young age and extensive lymphovascular invasion as high-risk disease. Currently, the decision on adding ovarian suppression remains somewhat empiric and as noted above a biomarker is critically needed. If no high-risk features are present, tamoxifen as single agent therapy remains standard of care. Therapy is recommended for at least five years. Extension to 10 years was evaluated in the ATLAS and aTTOMs trial (Table 2.2) and was shown to improve outcome [8, 16].

2.3.3.2   Postmenopausal Women

In postmenopausal women, the inclusion of an AI as adjuvant endocrine therapy is recommended. Current NCCN guidelines support the following: AI for 5 years; AI before or after 2–3 years of tamoxifen use; and AI as extended therapy after 5 years of tamoxifen. In patients unable to tolerate an AI, tamoxifen for at least 5 years with consideration of 10 years is recommended.

2.3.4   Duration of Therapy

HR-positive breast cancers are known to be at risk for late recurrences. Guidelines for 5 years of tamoxifen therapy stem from NSABP-B14, which showed a higher recurrence rate in patients with HR-positive node-negative breast cancer treated with 10 years of tamoxifen compared to 5 years of therapy [23]. Since then, several trials (Table 2.2) have shown a benefit of extending hormonal therapy to 10 years. The MA-17 trial showed a benefit in disease-free survival in patients who took letrozole therapy for a planned additional 5 years, compared to placebo, after 5 years of tamoxifen, especially in patients with node-positive breast cancers [13]. The aTTOM (adjuvant Tamoxifen: To Offer More?) and ATLAS (Adjuvant Tamoxifen: Longer Against Shorter) compared 5–10 years of tamoxifen. Both trials showed a reduced risk of recurrence and mortality with longer therapy, though this difference was not noted until 10 years following diagnosis [16, 17]. ATLAS showed a 3.7% absolute risk reduction with 10 years of tamoxifen compared to 5 years (21.4% vs. 25.1%). As expected, the risk of endometrial malignancies and venous thromboembolic events (VTEs) was increased with increased duration of tamoxifen. Overall these trials support either continuing tamoxifen for 10 years or switching to an aromatase inhibitor for 5 years following 5 years of tamoxifen.

Trials evaluating the continuation of AIs beyond 5 years (Table 2.2) have shown inconclusive results to date. The MA.17R [15] evaluated extending AI therapy for 10 years versus stopping at 5 years. Approximately 70% of patients had received tamoxifen for approximately 5 years prior to starting AI therapy. Results showed an added benefit of extended AI therapy to total 10 years in terms of contralateral breast cancer occurrence, but the overall effect on recurrence was modest. The NSABP B-42 [19, 20] trial enrolled postmenopausal women who have HR-positive cancers and had completed 5 years of hormonal therapy with either 5 years AI or tamoxifen followed by an AI for total 5 years. Patients were randomized for additional 5 years of letrozole or placebo therapy. The study, which included 3923 patients, did not show a statistically significant benefit in disease-free survival with an additional 5 years of letrozole (84.7%) versus placebo (81.3%). While there was no significant disease-free survival benefit, there was a significant improvement in breast-cancer-free interval (BCFI) with a 29% reduction along with a 28% reduction in distant recurrence for patients randomized to extended therapy. There was a notable increase in arterial thrombotic events in patients on long-term letrozole but no significant increase in osteoporotic fractures.

The question still remains as to which patients truly benefit from extended endocrine therapy, especially as patients with low-risk, luminal A cancers have a low rate of recurrence beyond 5 years. In contrast, luminal B cancers continue to have a higher rate of recurrence up to 10 years following diagnosis. Molecular profiling, as noted above, may help to determine which patients need extended therapy but require further validation. Overall, the decision to extend adjuvant therapy should be made with one-on-one discussion with the patient.

2.3.5   Male Breast Cancer

The majority of male breast cancers are HR-positive, and endocrine therapy is recommended to decrease the risk of recurrence. Retrospective studies and extrapolation from adjuvant endocrine studies provide the mainstay of evidence supporting this practice [12, 26]. Tamoxifen is the only agent that has been demonstrated to definitely decrease recurrence in male breast cancer. A retrospective study including 257 male patients with stage I to III breast cancer evaluated tamoxifen compared with AI therapy and showed that AI was associated with a poorer overall survival compared to tamoxifen [9]. Therefore, tamoxifen remains the adjuvant therapy of choice in males with HR-positive breast cancer.

2.3.6   Future Directions

Despite the success of endocrine therapy in decreasing recurrence from HR-positive early-stage breast cancer, women continue to experience recurrences, resulting in incurable metastatic disease. A number of agents have been shown to enhance the efficacy of endocrine therapy in patients with HR-positive metastatic disease and are now being evaluated in the early-stage setting. The SWOG 1207 trial (NCT01674140) randomizes patients with early-stage HR-positive breast cancer to endocrine therapy alone or with everolimus. The PALbociclib CoLlaborative Adjuvant (PALLAS) Study (NCT02513394) is evaluating the addition of palbociclib to endocrine therapy in patients with early-stage HR-positive breast cancer. Other trials are evaluating the other CDK inhibitors in the early-stage setting.

2.4 Conclusions

Adjuvant endocrine therapy has been shown to decrease breast cancer recurrence and decrease breast cancer mortality, in patients with early-stage HR-positive breast cancer. In premenopausal women, tamoxifen remains standard for the majority of patients, with ovarian suppression and endocrine therapy being reserved for patients with higher-risk cancers. In postmenopausal women, AIs are the treatment of choice, although efficacy is only modestly improved compared with tamoxifen. Therapy is current recommended for at least 5 years; however, an undefined subset of patients may benefit from longer duration of therapy. Molecular profiling assays provide additional information regarding risks of recurrence and potential benefit with adjuvant chemotherapy in HR-positive early-stage breast cancer. Future studies are currently evaluating the addition of agents that have been shown to enhance endocrine therapy in the metastatic setting to standard endocrine therapy. These offer the possibility of further improving outcome for patients with HR-positive breast cancer.

References

1. Albain KS et al (2010) Prognostic and predictive value of the 21-gene recurrence score assay in postmenopausal women with node-positive, oestrogen-receptor-positive breast cancer on chemotherapy: a retrospective analysis of a randomised trial. The Lancet Oncology 11(1): 55–65
2. Anonymous (2010) Pathologists' guideline recommendations for immunohistochemical testing of estrogen and progesterone receptors in breast cancer. Breast Care (Basel) 5(3):185–187
3. Breast International Group (BIG) 1-98 Collaborative Group, Thürlimann B et al (2006) A comparison of letrozole and tamoxifen in postmenopausal women with early breast cancer. N Engl J Med 353(26):2747–2757. Erratum in: N Engl J Med 2006 May 18, 354(20):2200
4. Buus R et al (2016) Comparison of EndoPredict and EPclin with Oncotype DX recurrence score for prediction of risk of distant recurrence after endocrine therapy. J Natl Cancer Inst 108(11)
5. Cardoso F et al (2016) MINDACT investigators. 70-gene signature as an aid to treatment decisions in early-stage breast cancer. N Engl J Med 375(8):717–729
6. Chia SK et al (2012) A 50-gene intrinsic subtype classifier for prognosis and prediction of benefit from adjuvant tamoxifen. Clin Cancer Res 18(16):4465–4472. Epub 2012 June 18

7. Coombes R et al (2004) Intergroup exemestane study. A randomized trial of exemestane after two to three years of tamoxifen therapy in postmenopausal women with primary breast cancer. N Engl J Med 350(11):1081–1092
8. Davies C et al (2013) Adjuvant tamoxifen: longer against shorter (ATLAS) collaborative group. Long-term effects of continuing adjuvant tamoxifen to 10 years versus stopping at 5 years after diagnosis of oestrogen receptor-positive breast cancer: ATLAS, a randomised trial. Lancet 381(9869):805–816
9. Eggeman H et al (2013) Adjuvant therapy with tamoxifen compared to aromatase inhibitors for 257 male breast cancer patients. Breast Cancer Res Treat 137(2):465–470. Epub 2012 Dec 9
10. Early Breast Cancer Trialists' Collaborative Group (EBCTCG) (2005) Effects of chemotherapy and hormonal therapy for early breast cancer on recurrence and 15-year survival: an overview of the randomised trials. Lancet 365(9472):1687–1717
11. Fisher B et al (1996) Five versus more than five years of tamoxifen therapy for breast cancer patients with negative lymph nodes and estrogen receptor-positive tumors. J Natl Cancer Inst 88(21):1529–1542
12. Giordano S et al (2005) Adjuvant systemic therapy for male breast carcinoma. Cancer 104 (11):2359
13. Goss P et al (2003) A randomized trial of letrozole in postmenopausal women after five years of tamoxifen therapy for early-stage breast cancer. N Engl J Med 349(19):1793–1802
14. Goss PE et al (2013) Exemestane versus anastrozole in postmenopausal women with early breast cancer: NCIC CTG MA.27–a randomized controlled phase III trial. J Clin Oncol. 2013 Apr 10;31(11):1398–1404
15. Goss P et al (2016) Extending aromatase-inhibitor adjuvant therapy to 10 years. N Engl J Med 375(3):209–219
16. Gray R et al, aTTom Collaborative Group (2013) aTTom: long-term effects of continuing adjuvant tamoxifen to 10 years versus stopping at 5 years in 6,953 women with early breast cancer. J Clin Oncol 31(18_suppl):5–5
17. Howell A et al, ATAC Trialists' Group (2005) Results of the ATAC (Arimidex, Tamoxifen, Alone or in Combination) trial after completion of 5 years' adjuvant treatment for breast cancer. Lancet 365(9453):60–62
18. Kaufmann M et al (2007) Improved overall survival in postmenopausal women with early breast cancer after anastrozole initiated after treatment with tamoxifen compared with continued tamoxifen: the ARNO 95 study. J Clin Oncol 25(19):2664–2670. Epub 2007 June 11
19. Mamounas E et al (2006) NSABP B-42: a clinical trial to determine the efficacy of five years of letrozole compared with placebo in patients completing five years of hormonal therapy consisting of an aromatase inhibitor (AI) or tamoxifen followed by an AI in prolonging disease-free survival in postmenopausal women with hormone receptor-positive breast cancer. Clin Breast Cancer 7(5):416–421
20. Mamounas E et al (2016) A randomized, double-blinded, placebo-controlled clinical trial of extended adjuvant endocrine therapy (tx) with letrozole (L) in postmenopausal women with hormone-receptor (+) breast cancer (BC) who have completed previous adjuvant tx with an aromatase inhibitor (AI): results from NRG Oncology/NSABP B-42 SABCS 2016, Abstract S1–05
21. Mamounas E et al (2010) Association between the 21-gene recurrence score assay and risk of locoregional recurrence in node-negative, estrogen receptor-positive breast cancer: results from NSABP B-14 and NSABP B-20. J Clin Oncol 28(10):1677–1683
22. Pagani O et al (2014) Adjuvant exemestane with ovarian suppression in premenopausal breast cancer. N Engl J Med 371(2):107–118
23. Paik S et al (2004) A multigene assay to predict recurrence of tamoxifen-treated, node-negative breast cancer. N Engl J Med 351(27):2817–2826
24. Paik S et al (2006) Gene expression and benefit of chemotherapy in women with node-negative, estrogen receptor-positive breast cancer. J Clin Oncol 24(23):3726–3734

25. Province et al (2014) CYP2D6 genotype and adjuvant tamoxifen: meta-analysis of heterogeneous study populations. Clin Pharmacol Ther 95(2):216–227
26. Ribeiro G et al (1992) Adjuvant tamoxifen for male breast cancer (MBC). Br J Cancer 65 (2):252
27. Sgroi D et al (2016) Assessment of the prognostic and predictive utility of the Breast Cancer Index (BCI): an NCIC CTG MA.14 study. Breast Cancer Res 18:1
28. Sorlie T et al (2003) Repeated observation of breast tumor subtypes in independent gene expression data sets. Proc Natl Acad Sci U S A 100(14):8418–8423
29. Sparano J et al (2015) Prospective validation of a 21-gene expression assay in breast cancer. N Engl J Med 373(21):2005–2014

Breast Cancer Screening: The Debate that Never Ends

3

Sarah M. Friedewald

Contents

Abstract

Screening mammography has been shown to decrease breast cancer deaths through randomized controlled trials. However, there remains significant debate surrounding the most appropriate time to commence screening and the optimal screening interval. Several national organizations have recently updated their guidelines by reanalyzing the published data. Interestingly, each organization has come to different conclusions regarding their recommendation for breast cancer screening in the average risk woman. Three of the main organizations that issue guidelines for breast cancer screening in the United States are reviewd in this chapter.

Keywords

Screening · Mammography · Randomized controlled trials · Breast imaging

S. M. Friedewald (✉)
Northwestern University, Feinberg School of Medicine, Chicago, IL, USA
e-mail: sarah.friedewald@nm.org

© Springer International Publishing AG 2018
W. J. Gradishar (ed.), *Optimizing Breast Cancer Management*, Cancer Treatment and Research 173, https://doi.org/10.1007/978-3-319-70197-4_3

3.1 Introduction

Eight randomized controlled trials have been performed evaluating the role of screening mammography in breast cancer mortality. Seven of the eight trials demonstrated reduction in breast cancer deaths when women were screened with a relative rate of breast cancer death ranging from 0.68 to 1.09 and an overall reduction by 24% [1–3]. However, despite this benefit, screening mammography demonstrates varying sensitivities, largely related to patient's breast density and age. This has been specifically studied by the Breast Cancer Surveillance Consortium (BCSC), a network of seven different breast imaging registries in the USA that collects information on over 2.3 million women who have attended screening mammography [4]. According to the BCSC data, sensitivities of mammography range from approximately 57% in women with dense breasts to nearly 93% in women with fatty breasts [5]. Therefore, despite significant effectiveness in detecting cancer and preventing breast cancer deaths, mammography has been a focus of criticism. Concerns regarding the lack of sensitivity of mammography are accompanied by the resulting anxiety for patients, unnecessary procedures, and increased costs for the health care system.

To complicate matters further, varying intervals of screening in the randomized trials and ages at which patients commenced their screening regimen were used. Therefore, standard recommendations for screening in the USA have been debated over the years and recently reevaluated. Many health care providers look to organizations for guidance such as the United States Preventive Services Task Force, American Cancer Society, and the National Comprehensive Care Network that issue screening mammography guidelines. The recommendations of these major organizations will be reviewed in this chapter.

3.2 United States Preventive Services Task Force (USPSTF)

The USPSTF is an independent volunteer panel of 16 members that specialize in prevention and primary care. The Task Force makes evidence-based recommendations about clinical preventive services. Since 1998 the Agency for Healthcare Research and Quality (AHRQ) has been authorized by the United States Congress to administer support to the Task Force. Each year the Task Force determines gaps in research and recommends areas that need attention [6]. The Task Force systematically reviews the literature and develops recommendations that take into consideration the net benefit of the intervention and the certainty of the benefit [7]. Standardized grades are assigned to the specific preventive service being evaluated and include the balance of the benefits versus the risks. Grades "A" and "B" signify that the service demonstrates a net benefit and is recommended. A grade of "C" denotes that the service is beneficial for some populations but should be based on professional judgement. The USPSTF recommends against providing a service when the service is given a grade "D". Finally, a grade of "I" suggests that there is insufficient evidence that there is a benefit to the reviewed service [8].

Historically, mammography screening was recommended by the USPSTF every 1–2 years for women aged 40 and older. However, the breast cancer screening recommendations were changed significantly in 2009 by the USPSTF and published in the Annals of Internal Medicine [9]. In this updated guideline, the USPSTF recommended biennial screening for women aged 50–74 years designating this a grade "B". Starting mammography prior to age 50 was given a "C" grade to suggest that only selected individuals should be receiving this service, siting that due to the low incidence of breast cancer in this age group, the relative risks associated with screening outweighed the benefits of lives saved. These risks included psychological harms, unnecessary imaging tests and biopsies in women without cancer, and inconveniences associated with false positives. Even more controversial was the recommendation against teaching self-breast examination. This was largely because of the high false positive rate associated with patients seeking breast imaging because of palpated abnormalities [9].

Interestingly, no new screening trials influenced the change in recommendations. However, updated information from one of the randomized control trials and use of modeling information from Cancer Intervention and Surveillance Modelling Network (CISNET) was incorporated into the new recommendations. The net benefit of mammography was determined to be greatest in women between ages 60 and 69 and that screening women from ages 50 to 69 provided a 17% reduction in mortality. The benefit for women in their 40s was smaller, and the risks associated with screening were greater in this age group, largely because of the larger number of women needed to be invited to screening to prevent one cancer death [10]. For older women, there were not enough data to support screening women past the age of 74 with little certainty about the benefits.

The change in recommendation from screening women yearly in their 40s to every other year beginning at age 50 was criticized. Some pointed out that no oncologists, radiologists, surgeons, or experts involved in breast cancer care were involved in the decision making. Additionally, the recommendations were based on data dating back to 1963 rather than gathering new information about screening. Digital mammography at this point largely had replaced film mammography, and therefore, it was felt that these recommendations were based on outdated technology. It was also argued that age 50 was an arbitrary threshold for commencing screening and that there are no data to support this change [11].

The recommendation to support biennial screening also was subject to criticism. The USPSTF concluded that the risks would be cut in half if patients were screened every other year but greater than two-year intervals would decrease the benefits by too much. However, critics claim that screening every other year decreases the opportunity to identify cancers at an earlier stage, the time when it is most curable. The longer the screening interval, the less effective the screening becomes. Opponents to the USPSTF updated recommendations also sited that optimal screening should be ½ the sojourn time, defined as the time which is a cancer is detected before it becomes clinically evident. Using a median doubling time of breast cancer cells of 130 days, it is estimated that the mean sojourn time for invasive breast cancer is 1.7 years before it becomes clinically palpable at 15 mm

[12, 13]. Therefore, screening at yearly intervals increases the likelihood that a cancer will be detected before it becomes palpable.

Finally, the uncertainties of overdiagnosis which was felt to be real, but unmeasured was a concern. Overdiagnosed malignancies are a subset of cancers that would have never harmed a woman during her lifetime had they remained undetected by mammography. However, it is impossible at the time of diagnosis to determine which cancers will become problematic. Therefore, all newly diagnosed breast cancers are currently treated with the assumption that they are lethal. Unfortunately, as a consequence, women who have indolent cancers will receive unnecessary surgery and other forms of treatment.

The true frequency of overdiagnosis from screening mammography is highly debated and very difficult to measure. Estimates vary widely from 0 to 50%. The most reliable way to estimate the frequency of overdiagnosis is to examine randomized controlled trials. Theoretically, if two randomized groups are truly equivalent and there is no overdiagnosis, the same number of cancers should be detected in both groups. In this scenario, those undergoing screening would have their cancers detected earlier compared to the control group. In the Malmo trial, screening detected approximately 10% more cancers than in the control group at 15 years of follow-up suggesting 10% overdiagnosis [14]. Two other randomized control trials (Two County and Gothenburg Trials) estimated even lower rates of overdiagnosis at 1% [15]. Finally, autopsy studies can be used as an estimate of disease burden. One study demonstrated 1.3% invasive breast cancer and 8.9% ductal carcinoma in situ (DCIS) identified at autopsy [16]. However, it is unlikely that overdiagnosed cancer exceeds what is identified at autopsy.

The frequency at which overdiagnosis occurs has not been well established, but it is inevitable that there will be some degree of overdiagnosis. The challenge is to find a way to distinguish clinically insignificant cancers detected at screening from those that, if untreated, would lead to death.

The USPSTF further updated their recommendations in 2016 which emphasized individualized decision making concluding that women who wished to be screened earlier than 50 should have the option to do so. The USPSTF states specifically, "The decision to start screening mammography in women prior to age 40 years should be an individual one. Women who place a higher value on the potential benefit than the potential harms may choose to begin biennial screening between the ages of 40 and 49 years" [17]. The grade recommendations did not change from the 2009 update.

3.3   American Cancer Society (ACS)

The American Cancer Society (ACS) also recently updated their guidelines, published in the Journal of the American Medical Association (JAMA) in 2015 [18]. These new guidelines were a departure from the 2003 recommendations where the ACS recommended yearly screening beginning at age 40 for as long as a woman was in good health. They commissioned a systematic review of the literature which focused on the quality of the data and the balance of the benefits and risks of screening. Similar to the USPSTF, the ACS did not utilize any new data to suggest that screening was less beneficial and underscored the benefits/risk ratio in specific age groups, whereas previous recommendations focused solely on the benefits of screening. However, the ACS examined patients in 5 year age groups, rather than 10 year groups. It was determined that women aged 45–49 were not significantly different than 50–55 year old women regarding the 5 year absolute risk of breast cancer at 0.9–1.1%, respectively [19]. Therefore grouping women in their early 40s who have 5 year absolute breast cancer risk of 0.6% with women in their later 40s was not appropriate. The ACS also emphasized that their recommendations were for average risk women and that recommendations for higher risk women would be updated at a later date Average risk women were defined as women who did not have a personal history of breast cancer, did not have a genetic mutation predisposing the patient to breast cancer, nor have had radiation to the chest at a young age.

Additionally, levels of recommendations were incorporated into the guidelines. Specifically, the ASC delineated two different types of recommendations; strong recommendations which conveyed certainty about the benefits, whereas qualified recommendations suggested that there were definitely benefits with screening, but included the option for patient preferences and values associated with screening possibly leading to different decisions about screening regimens. This is the first time the ACS included shared decision making in their breast cancer screening guidelines.

The recommendations by the ACS include a strong recommendation to screen women beginning at age 45 yearly until age 54. Women aged 55 and older could transition to biennial screening or if preferred could continue yearly screening. Likewise, women in their early 40s should have the option of screening yearly. These latter two recommendations were both qualified, incorporating patient values and preferences [18]. The ACS outlined that cessation of screening should occur if the patient has a less than 10 year life expectancy which clarified and further defined the previous 2003 recommendation of "screening as long as the patient is in good health" [20].

Just as controversial as the USPSTF not recommending teaching self-breast examinations, the ACS concurs that clinical breast examination generates too many false positive examinations. Instead, their recommendation is to use the time to educate patients on the benefits and risks associated with screening.

3.4   National Comprehensive Cancer Network (NCCN)

The NCCN guidelines were also recently updated in 2016 and are more consistent with the original ACS recommendations. Patients are stratified based on breast cancer risk. A patient at increased risk is defined by the NCCN as having a prior history of breast cancer, prior radiation to the chest before the age of 30, or if the patient has a greater than or equal to 1.7% 5 year risk or >20% lifetime risk of developing breast cancer. If the patient is at average risk of developing breast cancer, then annual screening is recommended beginning at age 40. Breast self-awareness is also included in their recommendations with the footnote stating "Women should be familiar with their breasts and promptly report changes to their health care provider" [21]. Therefore, the NCCN guidelines do not recommend for or against self-breast examination, but do specify the definition of an adequate examination including, supine and upright examination and inclusion of the axilla and clavicular regions. The NCCN also encourages consideration of life expectancy, specifically, women who may have significant comorbidities, although do not define a definitive age to cease screening.

Despite the fact that all of the randomized control trials utilized film mammography, the Digital Mammography Imaging Screening Trial (DMIST) demonstrated that digital mammography was superior for detection of breast cancer in women with dense breasts and women who were premenopausal [22]. Therefore, the NCCN guidelines include digital mammography as an acceptable modality for screening. Additionally, the NCCN guidelines recommend consideration of digital breast tomosynthesis (DBT), a newer mammographic screening technique FDA approved in 2011. DBT has been shown to not only improve cancer detection, but also decrease the false positives associated with screening, thereby improving upon the two main criticisms of standard mammography [23]. However, as with digital mammography, long-term outcomes of patients screened with DBT have not been studied. Therefore, surrogate markers are used to determine performance improvement such as cancer detection rate and decrease of false positive recalls. Inclusion of DBT in the screening guidelines is contrary to the USPSTF who claimed there was insufficient evidence to support the use of DBT as a primary screening tool or the use of supplemental screening modalities such as ultrasound or MRI.

3.5   Discussion

There is no debate that screening patients with mammography saves lives. All of the major guidelines agree that the most lives are saved when patients are screened yearly beginning at age 40. However recently, concern regarding the value of this service has been incorporated into the guidelines with particular attention to patient anxiety, inconveniences of additional testing in patients without breast cancer, and the associated costs with the false positive examinations. Therefore, emphasis is placed on communication of the benefits and risks to the patients by the providers. Patients are now playing a larger role in their care and can make shared decisions regarding their screening regimens.

References

1. Hendrick RE, Helvie MA (2012) Mammography screening: a new estimate of number needed to screen to prevent one breast cancer death AJR. Am J Roentgenol 198(3):723–728
2. Miller AB, Wall C, Baines CJ et al (2014) Twenty five year follow-up for breast cancer incidence and mortality of the Canadian National Breast Screening Study: randomised screening trial. BMJ 348:g366
3. Tabár L, Fagerberg G, Duffy SW et al (1989) The Swedish Two-County Trial of mammographic screening for breast cancer: recent results and calculation of benefit. J Epidemiol Commun Health 43:107–114
4. Breast cancer Surveillance Consortium Accessed at https://breastscreening.cancer.gov on 19 July 2017
5. Kerlikowske K et al (2015) Identifying women with dense breasts at high risk for interval cancer: a cohort study identifying women with dense breasts at high risk for interval cancer. Ann Intern Med 162(10):673–681
6. U. S. Preventive Services Task Force. About the USPSTF. Accessed at https://www.uspreventiveservicestaskforce.org/Page/Name/about-the-uspstf on 22 July 2017
7. Bibbins-Domingo K, Whitlock E, Wolff T, et al (2017) Developing recommendations for evidence-based clinical preventive services for diverse populations: methods of the U.S. preventive services task force. Ann Intern Med. 166(8):565–571
8. United States Preventive Services Task Force. grade definitions. Accessed at https://www.uspreventiveservicestaskforce.org/Page/Name/grade-definitions on 22 July 2017
9. U.S. Preventive Services Task Force (2009), screening for breast cancer: U.S. preventive services task force recommendation statement. Ann Intern Med 151:716–726
10. Mandelblatt JS, Cronin KA, Bailey S et al (2009) Effects of mammography screening under different screening schedules: model estimates of potential benefits and harms. Ann Intern Med 151:738–747
11. Kopans DB (2005) Informed Decision Making: Age of 50 is arbitrary and has no demonstrated influence on breast cancer screening in women. AJR 185:176–182
12. Michaelson JS, Satija S, Moore R (2003) Estimates of breast cancer growth rates and sojourn time from screening database information. J Women's Imaging 5:11–19
13. Michaelson JS, Satija S, Moore R (2003) Estimates of the sizes at which breast cancers become detectable on mammographic and clinical grounds. J Women's Imaging 5:3–10
14. Zackrisson S, Andersson I, Janzon L, Manjer J, Garne JP (2006) Rate of over-diagnosis of breast cancer 15 years after end of Malmö mammographic screening trial: follow-up study. BMJ 332(7543):689–692
15. Tabár L, Fagerberg G, Duffy SW et al (1989) The Swedish Two-County Trial of mammographic screening for breast cancer: Recent results and calculation of benefit. J Epidemiol Community Health 43:107–114
16. Welch HG, Black WC Using autopsy series to estimate the disease "reservoir" for ductal carcinoma in situ of the breast: how much more breast cancer can we find? Ann Intern Med 1 Dec 1997 127(11):1023
17. United States Preventive Services Task Force. Breast Cancer: screening Accessed at https://www.uspreventiveservicestaskforce.org/Page/Document/UpdateSummaryFinal/breast-cancer-screening1 on 22 July 2017
18. Oeffinger KC, Fontham ET, Etzioni R (2015) Breast cancer screening for women at average risk: 2015 guideline update from the american cancer society. JAMA 314(15):1599–1614
19. Howlander N, Noone A, Krapcho M et al SEER Cancer Statistics Review, 1975–2012. Bethesda, MD: National Cancer Institute; http://seer.cancer.gov/csr/1975_2012/, based on November 2014 SEER data submission, posted to the SEER web site, April 2015

20. Smith RA, Saslow D, Sawyer KA et al (2003) American Cancer Society guidelines for breast cancer screening: update 2003. CA Cancer J Clin 53(3):141–169
21. National Comprehensive Cancer Network Breast Cancer Screening and Diagnosis (2017) V. 1.2017. Accessed at https://www.nccn.org/professionals/physician_gls/pdf/breast-screening.pdf on 24 July 2017
22. Pisano ED, Gatsonis C, Hendrick E et al (2005) Diagnostic performance of digital versus film mammography for Breast-cancer screening. N Engl J Med 353:1773–1783
23. Friedewald SM, Rafferty EA, Rose SL et al (2014) JAMA 311(24):2499–2507

Management of the Axilla in Early Breast Cancer

Monica G. Valero and Mehra Golshan

Contents

M. G. Valero · M. Golshan (✉)
Department of Surgery, Brigham and Women's Hospital, 75 Francis Street,
Boston, MA 02115, USA
e-mail: mgolshan@bwh.harvard.edu

M. G. Valero
e-mail: mvalero@partners.org

M. Golshan
Breast Oncology Program, Susan F. Smith Center for Women's Cancer,
Dana-Farber/Brigham and Women's Cancer Center, Boston, MA, USA

© Springer International Publishing AG 2018
W. J. Gradishar (ed.), *Optimizing Breast Cancer Management*, Cancer Treatment
and Research 173, https://doi.org/10.1007/978-3-319-70197-4_4

Abstract

Management of the axilla in early breast cancer patients has significantly evolved in the last several decades. With the arrival of the sentinel lymph node biopsy, surgical practice for axillary staging in patients with early breast cancer has become gradually less invasive and formal axillary lymph node dissection has been confined to selected patients. Over the last two decades, evidence from randomized clinical trials have allowed for the de-escalation of axillary surgery in the management of early stage breast cancer. Advances in the staging and treatment of the axilla constitute a key component in determining initial surgical planning and therapeutic strategies in the treatment of early breast cancer. This chapter provides an updated review on the history, evolution, and current practices for axillary management in patients with early breast cancer, with particular attention to the surgical recommendations and controversial scenarios of the evolving management of the axilla.

Keywords
Sentinel lymph node biopsy · Axillary staging

4.1 Introduction

Significant advances over the last several decades have been reported in the multidisciplinary management of patients with breast cancer. Advances such as screening mammography, the development of targeted and less toxic systemic therapy, improved radiation therapy planning and dosing, the adoption of breast-conserving surgery (BCS), and the use of sentinel lymph node biopsy (SLNB) have influenced and improved the care and outcomes of patients with breast cancer.

The surgical treatment of the breast and the axilla has evolved from the radical axillary lymph node dissection (ALND) to the less invasive SLNB, and in some cases, even forgoing axillary staging altogether. SLNB has become the standard approach for axillary staging in patients with early-stage breast cancer, providing accurate staging with decreased rates of lymphedema and morbidity, and improved quality of life when compared to an ALND [1]. Dr. Donald Morton first introduced the concept for SLNB in 1992, which consisted of a minimally invasive procedure for detection of occult lymph node metastasis in melanoma surgery. Since this development, the importance of regional lymph nodes status and the use of SLNB in early breast cancer became an area of significant debate for providers in the field. Despite this early discovery, ALND continued as the standard of care until the twenty-first century when SLNB was validated and incorporated into practice for surgical management of the axilla [1].

4.2 History of Axillary Surgery

There have been significant advances in the surgical and clinical management of axillary dissection in breast cancer. It started with the introduction of the radical mastectomy by Halsted at the end of the nineteenth century [2]. Subsequently, in the 1930s, D.H Patey of the UK popularized the modified radical mastectomy (MRM), which focused on sparing the pectoral muscle while removing the breast tissue and axillary content (I–III). This operation eventually replaced the radical mastectomy when long-term follow-up not only failed to demonstrate breast cancer recurrence when preserving the pectoral muscles, but also showed no difference in survival outcomes compared with radical mastectomy [3].

These findings led clinicians to question the impact of local or regional control on overall survival. The National Surgical and Adjuvant Breast Project (NSABP) addressed these questions, and Dr. Bernard Fischer postulated that breast cancer was a systemic disease at presentation. One of the initial trials conducted by the NSABP—the NSABP B-04 [4]—was a randomized clinical trial that aimed to address the controversy over the ideal management of ALND. Conducted between 1971 and 1974, the study included 1079 patients with operable invasive breast cancer and clinically negative lymph nodes. These patients were randomized to one of three arms: (1) radical mastectomy, (2) total mastectomy without axillary dissection but with postoperative radiation, and (3) total mastectomy with a delayed axillary dissection only if patients developed clinically positive axillary nodes. An additional 586 patients with clinically positive lymph nodes were randomized to either radical mastectomy or total mastectomy without axillary surgery, but with postoperative radiation.

Based on 20 year of follow-up data, the B-04 trial demonstrated no survival advantage among both the node-negative treatment group and the node-positive treatment group; however, the trial was neither designed nor powered to address the question of axillary recurrence and survival. This trial also demonstrated the necessity of surgical lymph node dissection in identifying regional disease and the superiority of surgical lymph node dissection when compared with axillary radiation for local disease control among clinically node-positive patients. Yet, the results failed to show a significant survival advantage from removing occult positive nodes at the time of initial surgery or from the addition of radiation therapy [4, 5].

Despite these findings, surgical management did not change and ALND remained the standard of care. The lack of power to detect small survival benefit for those who had ALND was the critical factor behind this decision [4]. Critics of the study highlighted that, in the mastectomy-only group, many surgeons still included a large number of axillary nodes with the specimen [6–8].

Subsequently, the surgical treatment of the breast and the axilla moved toward a less radical intervention and the ALND was challenged by the introduction of SLNB. The concept for SLNB in breast cancer continued to develop. In 1993, Dr. David Krag and colleagues reported results of lymphatic mapping using technetium-99 to identify the first draining lymph node and lymphoscintigraphy was used as a confirmatory method. The authors concluded that the technique reliably localized the sentinel lymph node (SLN) of primary melanoma [9]. In 1994, Dr. Armando Giuliano and colleagues first described the use of SLNB in breast cancer patients using isosulfan blue dye [10]. Giuliano described it as an accurate method to obtain information about the axilla in clinically node-negative breast cancer patients.

Utilization of the combined blue dye and isotope mapping technique was first reported by Albertini et al. [11]. This theory was then replicated by Veronesi et al. [12] who performed SLNB in 163 consecutive patients using dual tracer (technetium-99 and lymphoscintigraphy) followed by complete axillary dissection. SLNB was able to accurately predict axillary disease in 97.5% of patients and in all patients with tumors less than 1.5 cm in diameter. Finally, in 2003 Veronesi et al. designed a randomized trial to compare SLNB and axillary dissection. They assigned patients with primary breast cancer and tumors less than 2 cm to either SLNB and axillary dissection or SLNB followed by axillary dissection only if metastases were found. This was the first trial to validate the accuracy of the SLNB as a predictor of the axillary status [1].

4.3   Technical Considerations of SLNB

A SLNB procedure consists of locating the sentinel lymph node through the use of an intradermal or subareolar injection at the tumor site with either a radiolabeled colloid (technetium-99m), blue dye (isosulfan blue, patent blue, or methylene blue), or a combination of both [13, 14].

Using the radiolabeled colloid technique, patients are injected with 0.5 ml or 0.5 mCi of filtered technetium-99m sulfur colloid (radiocolloid) into the skin, subdermally or in the peritumoral area of the breast, before surgery. Surgeons may perform a lymphoscintigram to document the drainage pattern of the breast lymphatics to the regional lymph nodes. During surgery, a gamma probe emits a signal that guides the surgeon to identify the sentinel node. The node with the greatest absolute counts can be defined as a radioactive node. It is generally accepted that all sentinel nodes with counts greater than 10% of the node with the highest absolute count should be removed. This guideline has been validated at Memorial Sloan Kettering Cancer Center and has shown that the rule of 10% correctly identifies 98.3% of positive nodes in patients with multiple sentinel nodes [15].

Surgeons utilizing the blue dye technique inject the blue dye intraoperatively into the breast and perform a gentle massage to help transfer the dye to the sentinel node. Sentinel nodes are identified by direct visualization of a blue lymphatic tract or blue-stained node. Different types of blue dye are used for SLNB: isosulfan blue dye, patent blue dye, or methylene blue dye. None of them is considered to be gold standard. Isosulfan blue dye, one of the first dyes approved by the US Food and Drug Administration (FDA) for use in SLNB, is a vital blue dye that is taken up by the lymphatic channels and trapped within the primary draining nodal basin. Isosulfan has a documented risk of allergic and anaphylactic reactions and can cause rash, hives, urticaria, pruritus, and hypotension. Allergic reactions, such as anaphylaxis, have been reported with the use of isosulfan, and series have shown incidence rates up to 2% [16]. The largest single institution review conducted by Memorial Sloan Kettering Cancer Center (2392 patients) described a 0.5% incidence of hypotension and a 1.6% incidence of allergic reactions to isosulfan blue dye [17]. To date, there are no recorded deaths related to isosulfan blue dye use. Alternatively, while methylene blue is equally effective, less costly, and has a lower risk of systemic reactions, it has been reported to have adverse reactions such as skin eruptions, rashes, subcutaneous tissue necrosis, and abscess formation [18–20].

The injection technique for SLNB has been examined in several studies, and multiple approaches have been described for injection of the blue dye, such as subdermal, intradermal, retroareolar, or peritumoral. Many studies suggest the superiority of intradermal injection compared with subdermal or deeper peritumoral breast injections [21, 22]. It is important to recognize that intradermal or subareolar injections of blue dye may cause tattooing of the nipple or skin, which may persist for months in patients undergoing breast conservation. In a patient undergoing a mastectomy, either an intradermal or subareolar injection of the blue dye is recommended. For a patient undergoing lumpectomy a retroareolar injection of the blue dye provides adequate localization without leaving the breast tattooed for an extended period of time.

Identification and removal of any suspicious nodes that are neither blue nor radioactive should be performed at the same procedure, as cancer-filled nodes may not take up dye or colloid. If the sentinel node is not identified, in general, an axillary node dissection should be performed, (level I and II ALND).

4.4 The SLN Era

4.4.1 Clinically Node-Negative Proof of Concept

To date, SLNB is routinely recommended in patients without clinical involvement of the axilla and spares patients from a complete axillary dissection if the sentinel node is negative. This concept is supported by several randomized controlled trials with long-term follow-up comparing axillary recurrence rates for SLNB and ALND.

Veronesi et al. [23] conducted a study comparing outcomes in 516 patients at a single institution randomized to SLNB alone versus SLNB plus routine completion ALND if the sentinel node was negative. At 10-years of follow-up, they reported no difference between the two groups with respect to disease-free survival (DFS); the overall survival (OS) was slightly higher in the SLNB alone group; however, this was not statistically significant.

The NSABP B-32 randomized controlled trial was subsequently designed to assess OS, DFS, rates of local recurrence, and associated morbidity in SLN-negative patients that underwent SLNB only versus ALND [24]. This study reported no significant difference in OS, DFS, and local recurrence between the two groups. Additionally, the study confirmed the low rate of regional recurrence after SLNB, which was previously reported in non-randomized studies. This proves that when the SLN is negative, SLNB alone is an appropriate, safe, and effective therapy for breast cancer patients with clinically negative lymph nodes.

4.4.2 Clinically Node Negative with Positive SLNB

The concept of the SLNB became adopted for the clinically node-negative patients with high sensitivity and specificity. The next question became whether having metastatic disease in the SLNB necessitates an ALND as the majority of patients with a positive SLN do not have additional nodes involved with disease. Three trials challenged this concept: Z0011, IBCSG 23-01, and AMAROS [25–27].

The American College of Surgeons Oncology Group (ACOSOG) Z0011 trial [25] was designed to compare the sentinel node biopsy for the clinically node-negative patient undergoing planned breast-conserving therapy with planned whole breast radiotherapy where women with one or two positive nodes were randomized to ALND versus no further axillary surgery. The Z0011 trial demonstrated no benefit in clearing axillary nodes when there was involvement of up to two sentinel nodes, and there was a very low axillary recurrence rate in patients not receiving completion ALND (0.9% after 6.3 years of follow-up). Therefore, the authors concluded that there is no difference in survival, local recurrence, or regional recurrence in patients with <2 positive sentinel nodes whether they receive ALND or not.

The IBCSG 23-01 [26] was a trial designed to determine whether axillary dissection could be omitted in patients with early breast cancer and one or more micrometastasis on SLNB. Patients were randomly assigned (in a 1:1 ratio) to either undergo axillary dissection or not to undergo axillary dissection. The primary outcome was DFS, and additional interests included axillary recurrence rates and complications. This trial reported no difference in DFS between axillary dissection versus no axillary dissection in patients with micrometastasis at a median follow-up of 5 years. Furthermore, they reported a low rate of disease recurrence in the patients with no axillary dissection (<1%) [23].

Furthermore, since the ACOSOG Z0011 and IBCSG 23-01 trials showed that patients with limited disease in the SLN treated with BCS, whole breast radiation, and adjuvant systemic therapy can be spared ALND without compromising locoregional control or survival, researchers now raised the question as to whether axillary radiotherapy provides comparable regional control with fewer side effects than axillary dissection.

Subsequently, studies such as the AMAROS trial [27], a multicenter randomized controlled trial designed to compare outcomes in patients with clinical T1–2 N0 primary breast cancer, found to have one or two positive nodes in SLNB who were randomly assigned to axillary radiotherapy or axillary lymph node dissection. The primary endpoint of the study was DFS; secondary endpoints included axillary recurrence rates and axillary surgical complications in the two groups of patients. The study confirmed that axillary lymph node dissection and axillary radiotherapy after a positive sentinel node biopsy provide excellent and comparable axillary control for patients with T1–2 primary breast cancer and a much lower rate of lymphedema in the axillary radiaiton arm.

4.5 Challenging Scenarios and Unanswered Questions

4.5.1 Prophylactic Mastectomy

In the modern era, prophylactic mastectomy has become an accepted procedure for patients with increased risk for developing breast cancer—such as BRCA-1 and BRCA-2 mutation carriers—as well as patients who are non-mutation carriers desiring symmetry, wishing to obviate the need for additional breast imaging, or experiencing anxiety about developing contralateral breast cancer. In a recent meta-analysis, the risk for nodal metastasis in this population was reported as 1.2%. SLNB is not a completely benign procedure with a small risk for developing lymphedema. Additionally, the risk of finding occult cancer is low: 3.2% for ductal carcinoma in situ (DCIS) and around 1.8% for invasive cancer, specifically 0.5% for invasive ductal carcinoma and 1.4% for invasive lobular carcinoma [28–30]. The majority of these cancers are at extremely low risk of harboring significant nodal disease, thus SLNB is not recommended routinely in patients undergoing prophylactic mastectomy.

4.5.2 Ductal Carcinoma in Situ

Patients with palpable DCIS or large areas of diffuse suspicious microcalcifications on core biopsy are at higher risk of having concomitant invasive disease. For the women undergoing breast-conserving surgery, SLNB is not currently recommended; however, it can be considered for patients considered high risk for having underlying associated invasive disease. The National Comprehensive Cancer Network (NCCN) updated the guidelines to recommend considering SLNB selectively for patients undergoing mastectomy. For patients considering mastectomy, these cases should be managed on an individual basis and merit a discussion with the multidisciplinary team as to whether information gleaned from a SLNB will impact further treatment decisions.

4.5.3 Multicentric Lesions

Based on the theory that multiple foci of cancer have different drainage patterns and have a false negative rate, it was initially thought that multicentric tumors were a contraindication for SLNB. Evidence suggests that breast fluid drains through the same afferent lymphatic channels to the same axillary sentinel node [31]. Additionally, the literature has reported success in identifying SLN with comparable false negative rates in patients with unifocal or multifocal lesions [32, 33]. Similar results have been reported in a five-year follow-up of a large series evaluating patients with multicentric breast cancer from a single institution. Patients underwent SLNB, and axillary dissection was performed only in cases of positive SLNB. From 138 patients with negative SLNB who did not receive axillary dissection, three patients (2.2%) developed axillary recurrence. Since axillary recurrence was infrequent in the group of negative SLNB, the recommendation states SLNB is an acceptable procedure for nodal staging in patients with multicentric breast disease and clinically negative axilla [6].

4.5.4 Elderly and Axillary Staging

Data suggest that there is an association between increasing age at diagnosis and the presence of more favorable cancer characteristics [34–36]. Therefore, researchers began investigating whether older patients with clinically negative nodes may benefit from a less aggressive axillary surgical approach.

The IBCGS trial 10-93 was one of the first randomized trials comparing axillary surgery versus no axillary surgery in patients older than 60 years old with clinically node-negative disease and adjuvant hormonal therapy. The results of this trial showed that avoiding axillary surgery altogether in this patient population transiently improved quality of life [36]. In certain elderly patients with clinically node-negative disease, SLNB can be omitted if the nodal status would not affect adjuvant treatment decisions [37]. In the CALGB 9343 trial, Hughes et al. [38] proved this concept with a 10-year follow-up study of women over 70 years old with clinically early stage node negative, estrogen receptor-positive breast cancer. Patients underwent lumpectomy and were randomized to receive either tamoxifen plus radiation or tamoxifen alone. The study results showed low rates of locoregional recurrence in both groups and no significant differences in time to distant metastasis, breast cancer-specific survival, or OS between the two groups. Six axillary recurrences were identified in the tamoxifen group and no axillary recurrence among the tamoxifen plus radiation group; however, just 244 received axillary staging, which represented one-third of the population.

The lack of consensus about management in elderly patients with breast cancer has led to practice variation with both over- and undertreatment of many patients. A study using the American College of Surgeons National Cancer Database, which represents approximately 80% of all newly diagnosed breast cancer, demonstrated significant variation in the performance of axillary staging in patients $\geq$ over

70 years old with early breast cancer across the USA [39]. Pesce et al. [39] showed that patients treated at academic institutions were 18.5% less likely to undergo axillary staging compared to practices in the community setting (OR 0.81, 95% CI 0.76–0.87).

Additionally, recent randomized clinical trials comparing axillary versus no axillary dissection in older patients (aged 65–80 years) with early breast cancer demonstrated a lack of benefit from axillary dissection after postoperative radiotherapy and adjuvant tamoxifen [40, 41]. While the omission of axillary staging in elderly patients with clinically negative axilla results in increased regional recurrence, it does not appear to impact survival [42].

Therefore, the NCCN recommends that axillary staging may be considered optional for older patients when the decision about a patient's need for adjuvant therapy is not affected by the results of the axillary dissection [43].

4.5.5 Prior Breast or Axillary Surgery

The majority of the large clinical trials excluded patients with prior breast or axillary surgery [12, 44]. Even though prior axillary surgery is often considered a contraindication for subsequent SLNB, there are limited data to support this concept. Retrospective single institution data suggest that SLNs may be identified even after prior surgeries in the breast or in the axilla [45, 46]. In addition, high success of SLNB after a surgical biopsy has been reported, regardless of the biopsy method or the excision volume removed before SLNB [47]. A study from Port et al. [48] demonstrated that a previous axillary operation (either an axillary dissection or previous successful or failed sentinel lymph node biopsy) did not prevent success of SLNB even when fewer than 10 nodes were removed during the previous procedure. The identification of the second SLNB was performed combining isotope mapping and dye techniques.

In a systematic review and meta-analysis of the literature including all studies on repeat SLNB in locally recurrent breast cancer, Maaskant-Braat et al. [50] reported the success rates of SLN identification by repeat axillary mapping based on previous axillary procedure and breast treatment. Overall, lymphatic mapping was successful in 405 of 572 patients (70.8%) (95% CI: 66.9–74.5). In patients with previous SLNB, lymphatic mapping was reported in 179 and was visualized in 148 of them (82.7%) (95% CI: 76.2–87.8). Among patients with previous ALND, lymphatic mapping was reported in 197 and visualized in 139 of them (70.6%) (95% CI: 63.6–76.7), which is significantly lower than after a previous SLNB ($P < 0.01$). The study also classified the lymphatic mapping data according to previous breast treatment. Among patients with previous breast-conserving therapy or lumpectomy, lymphatic mapping was recorded in 425 patients and was successful in 309 of them (72.7%) (95% CI: 68.2–76.8). Among patients with a previous mastectomy, lymphatic mapping was reported in 41 patients and successful in 31 of them (75.6%) (95% CI: 59.4–87.1) ($P =$ NS). The authors concluded that the longer the interval between the first and second lymphatic mapping in addition to the less invasive nature of the prior intervention lead to better results on reoperation after previous axillary or breast surgery. Therefore, unnecessary lymph node dissections may be avoided in selected groups of patients. These findings reinforced the updated clinical practice guideline to support the use of SLNB in patients who have undergone prior breast surgery [51].

4.5.6 Pregnancy

Breast cancer in pregnancy constitutes a challenging situation. Mammary gland changes associated with lactation as well as difficulty imaging pregnant patients can delay the diagnosis and treatment of breast cancer in this population. The role of SLNB in pregnant patients with early-stage breast cancer has been controversial. Initially, the recommendations from two consensus panels in 2001 and 2005 were against performing SLNB in pregnancy [51]. Subsequently, in 2006, an international panel accepted SLNB as an appropriate consideration in this population after informed discussion between surgeon and patient [52, 53]. The American Society of Clinical Oncology reported that there are insufficient data to change the 2005 recommendations specifying that pregnant patients should not undergo SLNB [54, 55]; however, other studies have reported that this procedure can be safely performed in pregnant patients [56, 57].

The potential concerns about using SLNB in pregnant patients include fetal harm from radiation exposure (radiocolloid use), fetal harm from possible teratogenicity of blue dyes, and fetal harm from maternal anaphylaxis to isosulfan blue dye, among others [51, 58, 59]. In terms of radiation exposure, the doses of injected radioactivity are relatively low with rapid clearance and uptake at the injection site and are surgically removed shortly after injection. This topic has been widely studied, and some authors have concluded that concern of radiation exposure should not preclude the use of SLNB during pregnancy [59–61]. Additionally, SLN procedures have been shown to lead to a negligible dose to the fetus of 0.014 mGy or less, which is much less than the National Council on Radiation Protection and Measurements' limit to a pregnant woman [62].

Dana-Farber/Harvard Cancer Center reported one of the largest studies of SLNB during pregnancy. The study included 81 women diagnosed with breast cancer during pregnancy between 1996 and 2013, and 47 were clinically node-negative patients who had surgery while pregnant: Twenty-five (53.2%) patients underwent SNB, 20 (42.6%) patients underwent upfront ALND, and two (4.3%) underwent no lymph node surgery. 99-Tc alone was used in 16 patients, methylene blue dye alone in seven patients, and two patients had unknown mapping methods. Mapping was successful in all patients. There were no SNB-associated complications. Among patients who underwent SNB, there were 25 live-born infants, of whom 24 were healthy, and one had cleft palate (in the setting of other maternal risk factors). The conclusion is that SLNB appears to be safe and accurate using either methylene blue or 99-Tc; however, numbers remain limited and further research is warranted [61].

4.6 Conclusion

The development, validation, practice, and evolution of SLNB have positively affected the treatment of early breast cancer. It provides accurate diagnosis and prognostic information in clinically node-negative early breast cancer patients and constitutes a paramount tool to advise patients and guide surgical and adjuvant treatments. In many cases, SLNB has replaced ALND and patients are spared the additional morbidity attributed to this procedure. The management for breast cancer will continue to evolve, and tailored treatment remains the goal. Axillary lymph node status will continue to have a critical role in both staging and in achieving locoregional control in selected breast cancer patients.

References

1. Veronesi U, Paganelli G, Viale G, Luini A, Zurrida S, Galimberti V et al (2003) A randomized comparison of sentinel-node biopsy with routine axillary dissection in breast cancer. N Engl J Med 349(6):546–553
2. Halsted WSI (1894) The results of operations for the cure of cancer of the breast performed at the Johns Hopkins Hospital from June, 1889, to January, 1894. Ann Surg 20(5):497–555
3. Adair F, Berg J, Joubert L, Robbins GF (1974) Long-term followup of breast cancer patients: the 30-year report. Cancer 33(4):1145–1150
4. Fisher B, Jeong JH, Anderson S, Bryant J, Fisher ER, Wolmark N (2002) Twenty-five-year follow-up of a randomized trial comparing radical mastectomy, total mastectomy, and total mastectomy followed by irradiation. N Engl J Med 347(8):567–575
5. Wickerham DL, Costantino JP, Mamounas EP, Julian TB (2006) The landmark surgical trials of the national surgical adjuvant breast and bowel project. World J Surg 30(7):1138–1146
6. Port ER, Tan LK, Borgen PI, Van Zee KJ (1998) Incidence of axillary lymph node metastases in T1a and T1b breast carcinoma. Ann Surg Oncol 5(1):23–27
7. Harris JR, Osteen RT (1985) Patients with early breast cancer benefit from effective axillary treatment. Breast Cancer Res Treat 5(1):17–21
8. Moore MP, Kinne DW (1996) Is axillary lymph node dissection necessary in the routine management of breast cancer? Yes. Important Adv Oncol 245–250
9. Alex JC, Weaver DL, Fairbank JT, Rankin BS, Krag DN (1993) Gamma-probe-guided lymph node localization in malignant melanoma. Surg Oncol 2(5):303–308
10. Giuliano AE, Kirgan DM, Guenther JM, Morton DL (1994) Lymphatic mapping and sentinel lymphadenectomy for breast cancer. Ann Surg 220(3):391–398. discussion 8–401
11. Albertini JJ, Lyman GH, Cox C, Yeatman T, Balducci L, Ku N et al (1996) Lymphatic mapping and sentinel node biopsy in the patient with breast cancer. JAMA 276(22): 1818–1822
12. Veronesi U, Galimberti V, Zurrida S, Pigatto F, Veronesi P, Robertson C et al (2001) Sentinel lymph node biopsy as an indicator for axillary dissection in early breast cancer. Eur J Cancer 37(4):454–458
13. Zakaria S, Hoskin TL, Degnim AC (2008) Safety and technical success of methylene blue dye for lymphatic mapping in breast cancer. Am J Surg 196(2):228–233
14. Blessing WD, Stolier AJ, Teng SC, Bolton JS, Fuhrman GM (2002) A comparison of methylene blue and lymphazurin in breast cancer sentinel node mapping. Am J Surg 184 (4):341–345

15. Chung A, Yu J, Stempel M, Patil S, Cody H, Montgomery L (2008) Is the "10% rule" equally valid for all subsets of sentinel-node-positive breast cancer patients? Ann Surg Oncol 15 (10):2728–2733

16. Newman LA (2004) Lymphatic mapping and sentinel lymph node biopsy in breast cancer patients: a comprehensive review of variations in performance and technique. J Am Coll Surg 199(5):804–816

17. Montgomery LL, Thorne AC, Van Zee KJ, Fey J, Heerdt AS, Gemignani M et al (2002) Isosulfan blue dye reactions during sentinel lymph node mapping for breast cancer. Anesth Analg 95(2):385–388 (table of contents)

18. Borgstein PJ, Meijer S, Pijpers R (1997) Intradermal blue dye to identify sentinel lymph-node in breast cancer. Lancet 349(9066):1668–1669

19. Stradling B, Aranha G, Gabram S (2002) Adverse skin lesions after methylene blue injections for sentinel lymph node localization. Am J Surg 184(4):350–352

20. Brady EW (2002) Sentinel lymph node mapping following neoadjuvant chemotherapy for breast cancer. Breast J. 8(2):97–100

21. Kern KA (1999) Sentinel lymph node mapping in breast cancer using subareolar injection of blue dye. J Am Coll Surg 189(6):539–545

22. Klimberg VS, Rubio IT, Henry R, Cowan C, Colvert M, Korourian S (1999) Subareolar versus peritumoral injection for location of the sentinel lymph node. Ann Surg 229(6): 860–864 (discussion 4–5)

23. Veronesi U, Viale G, Paganelli G, Zurrida S, Luini A, Galimberti V et al (2010) Sentinel lymph node biopsy in breast cancer: ten-year results of a randomized controlled study. Ann Surg 251(4):595–600

24. Krag DN, Anderson SJ, Julian TB, Brown AM, Harlow SP, Costantino JP et al (2010) Sentinel-lymph-node resection compared with conventional axillary-lymph-node dissection in clinically node-negative patients with breast cancer: overall survival findings from the NSABP B-32 randomised phase 3 trial. Lancet Oncol. 11(10):927–933

25. Giuliano AE, Hunt KK, Ballman KV, Beitsch PD, Whitworth PW, Blumencranz PW et al (2011) Axillary dissection vs no axillary dissection in women with invasive breast cancer and sentinel node metastasis: a randomized clinical trial. JAMA 305(6):569–575

26. Galimberti V, Cole BF, Zurrida S, Viale G, Luini A, Veronesi P et al (2013) Axillary dissection versus no axillary dissection in patients with sentinel-node micrometastases (IBCSG 23-01): a phase 3 randomised controlled trial. Lancet Oncol. 14(4):297–305

27. Donker M, van Tienhoven G, Straver ME, Meijnen P, van de Velde CJ, Mansel RE et al (2014) Radiotherapy or surgery of the axilla after a positive sentinel node in breast cancer (EORTC 10981-22023 AMAROS): a randomised, multicentre, open-label, phase 3 non-inferiority trial. Lancet Oncol. 15(12):1303–1310

28. Nagaraja V, Edirimanne S, Eslick GD (2016) Is sentinel lymph node biopsy necessary in patients undergoing prophylactic mastectomy? A systematic review and meta-analysis. Breast J. 22(2):158–165

29. Boughey JC, Khakpour N, Meric-Bernstam F, Ross MI, Kuerer HM, Singletary SE et al (2006) Selective use of sentinel lymph node surgery during prophylactic mastectomy. Cancer 107(7):1440–1447

30. Boughey JC, Attai DJ, Chen SL, Cody HS, Dietz JR, Feldman SM et al (2016) Contralateral prophylactic mastectomy (CPM) consensus statement from the American Society of Breast Surgeons: data on CPM outcomes and risks. Ann Surg Oncol 23(10):3100–3105

31. Jin Kim H, Heerdt AS, Cody HS, Van Zee KJ (2002) Sentinel lymph node drainage in multicentric breast cancers. Breast J. 8(6):356–361

32. Kumar R, Jana S, Heiba SI, Dakhel M, Axelrod D, Siegel B et al (2003) Retrospective analysis of sentinel node localization in multifocal, multicentric, palpable, or nonpalpable breast cancer. J Nucl Med 44(1):7–10

33. Tousimis E, Van Zee KJ, Fey JV, Hoque LW, Tan LK, Cody HS 3rd et al (2003) The accuracy of sentinel lymph node biopsy in multicentric and multifocal invasive breast cancers. J Am Coll Surg 197(4):529–535

34. Pierga JY, Girre V, Laurence V, Asselain B, Dieras V, Jouve M et al (2004) Characteristics and outcome of 1755 operable breast cancers in women over 70 years of age. Breast 13(5): 369–375

35. Diab SG, Elledge RM, Clark GM (2000) Tumor characteristics and clinical outcome of elderly women with breast cancer. J Natl Cancer Inst 92(7):550–556

36. International Breast Cancer Study G, Rudenstam CM, Zahrieh D, Forbes JF, Crivellari D, Holmberg SB et al (2006) Randomized trial comparing axillary clearance versus no axillary clearance in older patients with breast cancer: first results of International Breast Cancer Study Group Trial 10–93. J Clin Oncol 24(3):337–344

37. Mc CD, Gemignani ML (2016) Current management of the Axilla. Clin Obstet Gynecol 59(4):743–755

38. Hughes KS, Schnaper LA, Bellon JR, Cirrincione CT, Berry DA, McCormick B et al (2013) Lumpectomy plus tamoxifen with or without irradiation in women age 70 years or older with early breast cancer: long-term follow-up of CALGB 9343. J Clin Oncol 31(19):2382–2387

39. Pesce C, Czechura T, Winchester DJ, Huo D, Winchester DP, Yao K (2013) Axillary surgery among estrogen receptor positive women 70 years of age or older with clinical stage I breast cancer, 2004–2010: a report from the National Cancer Data Base. Ann Surg Oncol 20 (10):3259–3265

40. Martelli G, Boracchi P, Ardoino I, Lozza L, Bohm S, Vetrella G et al (2012) Axillary dissection versus no axillary dissection in older patients with T1N0 breast cancer: 15-year results of a randomized controlled trial. Ann Surg 256(6):920–924

41. Martelli G, Boracchi P, Orenti A, Lozza L, Maugeri I, Vetrella G et al (2014) Axillary dissection versus no axillary dissection in older T1N0 breast cancer patients: 15-year results of trial and out-trial patients. Eur J Surg Oncol 40(7):805–812

42. Liang S, Hallet J, Simpson JS, Tricco AC, Scheer AS (2016) Omission of axillary staging in elderly patients with early stage breast cancer impacts regional control but not survival: a systematic review and meta-analysis. J Geriatr Oncol 140–147

43. Gradishar WJ, Anderson BO, Balassanian R, Blair SL, Burstein HJ, Cyr A, et al (2017) Breast cancer, Version 2.2017: National Comprehensive Cancer Network; 6 Apr 2017. Available from: https://www.nccn.org/professionals/physician_gls/f_guidelines.asp

44. Viale G, Zurrida S, Maiorano E, Mazzarol G, Pruneri G, Paganelli G et al (2005) Predicting the status of axillary sentinel lymph nodes in 4351 patients with invasive breast carcinoma treated in a single institution. Cancer 103(3):492–500

45. Heuts EM, van der Ent FW, Kengen RA, van der Pol HA, Hulsewe KW, Hoofwijk AG (2006) Results of sentinel node biopsy not affected by previous excisional biopsy. Eur J Surg Oncol 32(3):278–281

46. Renaudeau C, Lefebvre-Lacoeuille C, Campion L, Dravet F, Descamps P, Ferron G et al (2016) Evaluation of sentinel lymph node biopsy after previous breast surgery for breast cancer: GATA study. Breast 28:54–59

47. Haigh PI, Hansen NM, Qi K, Giuliano AE (2000) Biopsy method and excision volume do not affect success rate of subsequent sentinel lymph node dissection in breast cancer. Ann Surg Oncol 7(1):21–27

48. Port ER, Fey J, Gemignani ML, Heerdt AS, Montgomery LL, Petrek JA et al (2002) Reoperative sentinel lymph node biopsy: a new option for patients with primary or locally recurrent breast carcinoma. J Am Coll Surg 195(2):167–172

49. Intra M, Trifiro G, Viale G, Rotmensz N, Gentilini OD, Soteldo J et al (2005) Second biopsy of axillary sentinel lymph node for reappearing breast cancer after previous sentinel lymph node biopsy. Ann Surg Oncol 12(11):895–899

50. Maaskant-Braat AJ, Voogd AC, Roumen RM, Nieuwenhuijzen GA (2013) Repeat sentinel node biopsy in patients with locally recurrent breast cancer: a systematic review and meta-analysis of the literature. Breast Cancer Res Treat 138(1):13–20

51. Lyman GH, Giuliano AE, Somerfield MR, Benson AB 3rd, Bodurka DC, Burstein HJ et al (2005) American Society of Clinical Oncology guideline recommendations for sentinel lymph node biopsy in early-stage breast cancer. J Clin Oncol 23(30):7703–7720

52. Loibl S, von Minckwitz G, Gwyn K, Ellis P, Blohmer JU, Schlegelberger B et al (2006) Breast carcinoma during pregnancy. International recommendations from an expert meeting. Cancer 106(2):237–246

53. Schwartz GF, Giuliano AE, Veronesi U, Consensus Conference C (2002) Proceedings of the consensus conference on the role of sentinel lymph node biopsy in carcinoma of the breast April 19 to 22, 2001, Philadelphia, Pennsylvania. Hum Pathol 33(6):579–589

54. Lyman GH, Somerfield MR, Bosserman LD, Perkins CL, Weaver DL, Giuliano AE (2016) Sentinel lymph node biopsy for patients with early-stage breast cancer: American Society of Clinical Oncology Clinical Practice Guideline Update. J Clin Oncol JCO2016710947 (Epub ahead of print)

55. Lyman GH, Temin S, Edge SB, Newman LA, Turner RR, Weaver DL et al (2014) Sentinel lymph node biopsy for patients with early-stage breast cancer: American Society of Clinical Oncology clinical practice guideline update. J Clin Oncol 32(13):1365–1383

56. Gentilini O, Cremonesi M, Trifiro G, Ferrari M, Baio SM, Caracciolo M et al (2004) Safety of sentinel node biopsy in pregnant patients with breast cancer. Ann Oncol 15(9):1348–1351

57. Gentilini O, Cremonesi M, Toesca A, Colombo N, Peccatori F, Sironi R et al (2010) Sentinel lymph node biopsy in pregnant patients with breast cancer. Eur J Nucl Med Mol Imaging 37(1):78–83

58. Toesca A, Luini A, Veronesi P, Intra M, Gentilini O (2011) Sentinel lymph node biopsy in early breast cancer: the experience of the European Institute of Oncology in Special Clinical Scenarios. Breast Care (Basel). 6(3):208–214

59. Spanheimer PM, Graham MM, Sugg SL, Scott-Conner CE, Weigel RJ (2009) Measurement of uterine radiation exposure from lymphoscintigraphy indicates safety of sentinel lymph node biopsy during pregnancy. Ann Surg Oncol 16(5):1143–1147

60. Morita ET, Chang J, Leong SP (2000) Principles and controversies in lymphoscintigraphy with emphasis on breast cancer. Surg Clin North Am 80(6):1721–1739

61. Gropper AB, Calvillo KZ, Dominici L, Troyan S, Rhei E, Economy KE et al (2014) Sentinel lymph node biopsy in pregnant women with breast cancer. Ann Surg Oncol 21(8):2506–2511

62. Pandit-Taskar N, Dauer LT, Montgomery L, St Germain J, Zanzonico PB, Divgi CR (2006) Organ and fetal absorbed dose estimates from 99mTc-sulfur colloid lymphoscintigraphy and sentinel node localization in breast cancer patients. J Nucl Med 47(7):1202–1208

Is DCIS Overrated?

5

Joshua Feinberg, Rachel Wetstone, Dana Greenstein
and Patrick Borgen

Contents

J. Feinberg
Department of Surgery, Maimonides Breast Center, Maimonides Medical Center,
Research Fellow, Oxford University, Oxford, England

R. Wetstone · D. Greenstein · P. Borgen (✉)
Department of Surgery, Maimonides Medical Center, Brooklyn, NY, USA
e-mail: PBorgen@maimonidesmed.org

© Springer International Publishing AG 2018
W. J. Gradishar (ed.), *Optimizing Breast Cancer Management*, Cancer Treatment
and Research 173, https://doi.org/10.1007/978-3-319-70197-4_5

Abstract

Ductal carcinoma in situ (DCIS), the noninvasive form of breast cancer (BC), comprises just over 20% of breast cancer cases diagnosed each year in the USA. Most patients are treated with local excision of the disease followed by whole breast radiation therapy. Total mastectomy is not an uncommon approach, and total mastectomy with a contralateral risk-reducing mastectomy has been on the rise in the past decade. In estrogen receptor-positive disease, patients are often offered endocrine ablative therapy with a selective estrogen receptor modulator or an aromatase inhibitor as both treatment and prevention. Local regional treatment options have no impact upon ultimate overall survival. Long-term survival rates are higher in patients with DCIS than with any other form of the disease. Are these strikingly high success rates a testament to effective treatment strategies or is there a significant subset of DCIS that was unlikely to ever progress to invasive ductal carcinoma? DCIS was not seen in the US prior to the advent of screening mammography. When compared to other countries, the USA has the highest utilization of screening mammography and the incidence rate of DCIS. Other lines of evidence include autopsy series examining the breast tissue of women who died of other causes, missed-diagnosis series and current retrospective reviews of DCIS, all align in support of the concept of DCIS as indolent in the majority of cases [3–14]. The evidence suggests that both patient and physician misconceptions about DCIS have led to overdiagnosis and over-treatment of DCIS. Recently, a gene expression profiling tool (12 gene assay, Oncotype DCIS) has emerged that shows considerable promise in predicting class in DCIS patients.

Keywords

Ductal carcinoma in situ · DCIS · Breast cancer · Breast cancer screening
Breast cancer genomic profiling

5.1　Introduction

In the past half-century, a number of very common human illnesses were treated based upon, what was eventually found to be, a flawed conceptualization of the underlying pathophysiology. For the general surgeon, no better example exists than the treatment of peptic ulcer disease (PUD). PUD was assumed to be, in the overwhelming majority of cases, due to excess acid production. Surgical careers were built on the fine tuning of the surgical treatment of PUD via an array of acid-reducing operative procedures. Vagotomy and antrectomy were deemed to be the most efficacious procedure while the highly selective vagotomy had far fewer complications. Helicobacter pylori was identified in 1982 by two Australian scientists, Robin Warren and Barry J. Marshall as a causative factor for ulcers. In their original paper, Warren and Marshall contended that most gastric ulcers and gastritis were caused by colonization with this bacterium, not by stress or spicy food as had been assumed before [1, 2]. The H. pylori hypothesis was initially poorly received, so in an act of self-experimentation, Marshall drank a Petri dish containing a culture of organisms extracted from a patient and five days later developed gastritis. His symptoms disappeared after two weeks, but he took antibiotics to kill the remaining bacteria at the urging of his wife since halitosis is one of the symptoms of infection. This experiment was published in 1984 in the Australian Medical Journal and is among the most cited articles from the journal. In 1997, the Centers for Disease Control and Prevention, with other government agencies, academic institutions, and industry, launched a national education campaign to inform health care providers and consumers about the link between H. pylori and ulcers. This campaign reinforced the news that ulcers are a curable infection and that health can be greatly improved and money saved by disseminating information about H. pylori. In 2005, the Karolinska Institute in Stockholm awarded the Nobel Prize in Physiology or Medicine to Dr. Marshall and his longtime collaborator Dr. Warren 'for their discovery of the bacterium Helicobacter pylori and its role in gastritis and peptic ulcer disease.'

Is it reasonable to compare the current treatment of ductal carcinoma in situ (DCIS) to the treatment of PUD? The answer is both yes and no. The causative agent in PUD was unknown prior to 1982, and the treatment assumptions were therefore innately flawed. The central issue with DCIS is the natural history of the disease and how our treatment strategies are based upon incorrect assumptions concerning DCIS as a putative obligate precursor to invasive duct carcinoma. Most DCIS was either never going to progress to invasive ductal disease or, at best, was predicted to progress at a slow rate that was not clinically meaningful. DCIS is a complex family of diseases that cannot be subcategorized using conventional clinical–pathologic features of the disease.

The authors of this chapter have two goals—(1) to examine the available evidence about the natural history of DCIS and (2) to explore current tools that may predict class in an attempt to subset DCIS and, logically, to match the treatment to the disease in hopes of avoiding over-treatment.

5.2 Anatomy

The breast consists of 13–24 segments, or lobes. Each lobe is based on a branching duct system leading from the terminal duct lobular units (TDLU) and collecting ducts via segmental and sub-segmental ducts to the major lactiferous ducts entering the nipple. The TDLU is the putative site of end-organ carcinogenesis in the breast. The segmental collecting systems do not communicate with one another, arguably a protective evolutionary advantage against catastrophic infection and the protection of the milk-producing apparatus. It is believed that the hormone-sensitive epithelial cells within the lobules are the major source of ductal carcinoma in situ (DCIS) of the breast. The neoplastic cells grow, fill, and increase the volume of the spaces bound by the basement membrane (on light microscopy). This process can lead to necrosis of tumor cells and subsequent formation of micro-calcification granules that are seen and investigated on mammography. Without micro-calcium deposits, it would not be possible to diagnose early DCIS lesions in the breast. Invasion of the basement membrane is not an inevitable event with DCIS. Even extensive cases of DCIS are truly unifocal in three dimensions and are usually confined to a single segment of the mammary duct system. The neoplastic cells can proliferate within the spaces that have been altered by benign proliferative diseases such as sclerosing adenosis, duct hyperplasia, radial scar, or even multiple papillomata. Atypical ductal hyperplasia (ADH) can be understood as very minimal low-grade DCIS that incompletely fills the spaces bounded by the basement membrane. Although ADH, atypical lobular hyperplasia, and lobular carcinoma in situ (LCIS) are associated with a general risk for later development of invasive mammary carcinoma, half of which occurs in the unaffected contralateral breast. It is reasonable to postulate that DCIS carries the same implications for future disease rather than as an obligate precursor to invasive mammary cancer.

5.3 Historical Perspectives on Natural History of DCIS

In 1919, James Ewing (1866–1943) of the Memorial Hospital for Cancer and Allied Diseases in New York City in his book on Neoplastic Diseases, classified breast carcinomas as adeno-carcinoma, ductal carcinoma, and acinar or alveolar carcinoma. On page 503, he illustrated the microscopy of a non-infiltrating 'large and small alveolar carcinoma.' The accompanying photomicrograph clearly shows an intraductal and in situ lobular carcinoma although those terms were never applied to the disease by Ewing. In 1932, Albert Broders (1885–1964) of the Mayo Clinic, Rochester, Minnesota, coined the term 'carcinoma in situ.'

Frank Foote (1911–1989) and Fred Stewart (1894–1991) at the Memorial Hospital for Cancer and Allied Diseases in New York City introduced the name 'LCIS.' Fundamentally they conceptualized LCIS as an obligate precursor to invasive lobular carcinoma. They were opposed in this view by leading pathologists such as Cushman Haagensen who argued that this lesion was not a precursor to invasive disease but rather was a marker of subsequent risk. Haagensen preferred to call this lesion lobular neoplasia an appellation that persists today in some centers. Foote and Stewart wrote that cancer of small lobular ducts and lobules could occur independently of the common breast cancer of the large ducts and that LCIS has the potential of invading and metastasizing. They correctly pointed out that lobular carcinoma in situ cannot be diagnosed clinically or on gross pathologic examination and went on to define LCIS as an incidental finding on excisions that have been performed for other conditions. The authors recommended simple mastectomy as the treatment, but admitted that wide local excision was also acceptable provided the patient is closely followed. After publication in 1950 of Stewart's AFIP Fascicle on Tumors of the Breast, lobular carcinoma in situ was generally recognized as a valid entity by pathologists and oncologists. This publication contains a clear description of ductal carcinoma in situ and may be the first place those words were specifically used to describe the condition in question—DCIS [15–23].

5.4   Ductal Carcinoma in Situ and Invasive Ductal Carcinoma

The most common type of breast malignancy, invasive ductal carcinoma (IDC), is the presumed endpoint in a progression initiated by a variety of benign fibrocystic mammary features including ductal hyperplasia (DH). The overwhelmingly appealing nature of a simple conceptual framework of a sequential progression from DH to IDC is opposed by epidemiological evidence showing that most ADH never becomes DCIS and most DCIS never becomes IDC [24–30].

Despite efforts to identify DCIS to IDC progression markers, relatively few useful prognostic biomarkers have been discovered to date. Genomic biomarker studies mainly applied gene expression microarrays or array copy genomic hybridization (aCGH) to lesions along the putative spectrum of progression. Predictably, many of these studies have identified highly similar gene copy number profiles and gene expression signatures within synchronous DCIS and IDC regions within the same breast. With the development of next-generation sequencing (NGS) technologies, investigators have begun to apply higher-resolution methods to study invasive ductal breast cancer-specific mutations and copy number events in patients with synchronous DCIS–IDC. Some of these studies have begun to identify both concordant and discordant mutations in patients with synchronous in situ and invasive ductal disease. However, these initial genomic studies faced several non-trivial technical obstacles, including low tumor purity, the unavailability of fresh-frozen tissues, and intra-tumor heterogeneity (ITH). Consequently, the genomic and molecular basis of invasion in DCIS remains poorly understood [31–48].

5.5   Clinical, Genomic, and Molecular Characteristics of DCIS

Histopathology of DCIS material using H&E staining has identified different distinct subtypes of DCIS; however, the clinical relevance of these findings has been called into doubt. Even the once ominous finding of central necrosis (comedo necrosis) has been called into question as clinically meaningful. The most common anatomic subclassifications of DCIS—solid, cribriform, comedo necrosis, micro-papillary—appear to have little association with neither natural history nor chance of recurrence.

Long-term follow-up studies of patients with DCIS have suggested a substantial difference in the progression of low-grade versus high-grade DCIS, with only 35% of low-grade DCIS patients progressing to IDC over 50 years, while 50% of high-grade DCIS progressed to IDC over 3 years. Previous reviews have discussed differences between low- and high-grade DCIS in detail. However, grade of DCIS is subject to pathologist bias and is difficult to reproduce in clinical trials. Studies that include both local and central assessment of grade in DCIS often reveal striking differences in grade assignment.

In the USA, DCIS is routinely queried for estrogen receptors (ERs) and progesterone receptors (PRs) to determine whether hormone receptor-based therapy should be recommended. Analysis of hormone receptor status shows that patients with ER+ and PR+ disease often have low-grade DCIS tumors which may be slightly less likely to progress than patients with ER− and PR− disease and high-grade tumors. While a new study showed that intra-tumor heterogeneity in the HER2 receptor was also associated with poor prognosis in DCIS patients, currently DCIS patients are not routinely tested for HER2 (ERBB2) amplification.

Low-grade DCIS is more often ER+/PR+/HER2−, with fewer copy number aberrations (CNAs) than high-grade DCIS. A high-grade DCIS has atypical nuclei and is more often ER− and PR−. High-grade DCIS usually has more genome-wide CNAs, including frequent events in 1q+, 5p+, 8p−, 8q+, 11q−, 13q−, 14q−, and 17q+ and focal amplifications on 6q22, 8q22, 11q13, 17q12, 17q22–24, and 20q13. Mutational markers of IDC include mutations in TP53 and PTEN (somatic not germline mutations), amplifications of chromosome 17 and 11q, and loss of PIK3CA mutations [49–56].

5.6   Models of Invasion

Conceptually, there are three fundamental models of invasion during progression of DCIS to IDC: (1) independent evolution; (2) evolutionary bottlenecks; and (3) multiclonal invasion (Fig. 5.1). The independent evolution model proposes that two different initiating cells (N1, N2) in normal breast tissue give rise separately to DCIS and IDC subpopulations. The independent lineage model is in distinct contrast to the direct lineage models (evolutionary bottlenecks and multiclonal evolution), which assume that a single normal breast cell (N1) gives rise to both DCIS and IDC populations. The main difference between the direct lineage models is that the evolutionary bottleneck model argues that a clone in the ducts is selected during invasion and migrates into adjacent tissue, forming the invasive tumor. In contrast, the multiclonal model posits that invasion occurs through escape of multiple clones from the duct, through a coordinated process or a stochastic escape after the degradation of basement membrane. In reality, it is likely that all three models may be correct within different DCIS tumors at different time points.

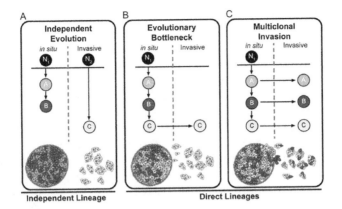

Fig. 5.1 Evolutionary models of invasion in DCIS. a Independent evolution model shows the in situ and invasive subpopulations evolving from independent lineages that originated from two different normal cells (N1, N2) in the breast. b Evolutionary bottleneck model shows the evolution of three clonal subpopulations from a single ancestral cell (N1), from which a single clone is selected during invasion and expands to form the invasive carcinoma. c Multiclonal invasion model shows the evolution of three clonal subpopulations from a single normal cell (N1) in the breast. In this model, all three clones escape the duct and co-migrate into the adjacent tissues to establish the invasive carcinoma. (Permission applied for: The Journal of Pathology Volume 241, Issue 2, pages 208–218, 27 NOV 2016 DOI:10.1002/path.4840 http://onlinelibrary.wiley.com/doi/10.1002/path.4840/full#path4840-fig-0002)

5.7   Incidence

In the USA, ductal carcinoma in situ (DCIS) accounts for about 20% of all breast cancer (BC), a tenfold increase from 2.8% of all cases in 1973. This increase is directly attributable to the popularization of screening mammography. The slope of the rate of increase in use of screening mammography from 1990 to 2000 matches the slope of the increasing incidence in DCIS almost exactly. Not surprisingly, the US incidence is three times higher than the rates in England and Switzerland. In 2007, digital mammography supplanted conventional analogue mammography and, predictably, the incidence of DCIS increased. Rejecting the idea that the radiation exposure received during conventional screening mammography might play a causative role in the development of DCIS, the only other logical explanation is that there is a non-trivial reservoir of DCIS that was either never going to progress to invasive breast cancer or, possibly, that the rate of progression to invasive disease is slow enough to be clinically meaningless.

5.8   Natural History of DCIS

The natural history of DCIS is poorly understood. Several different strategies have been applied to shed light on the natural history of DCIS beyond the inferences drawn from the screening mammography studies.

Several studies of misdiagnosis, wherein cases of DCIS were initially misdiagnosed as benign and therefore, were left alone in the breast, provide insight. Page et al. conducted a retrospective study and found that 28 subjects out of 11,760 cases who were initially diagnosed with benign breast disease, actually contained DCIS. Only 9/28 (32%) patients developed any form of invasive breast cancer for up to 31 years after biopsy alone. Betsill et al. reported a long-term follow-up study of patients diagnosed with low-grade papillary intraductal carcinomas that were initially missed, who were treated by biopsy alone. Forty percent of these patients were alive free of invasive breast cancer 9.7 years after diagnoses. Additionally, Rosen et al. performed a retrospective review of thousands of biopsies and found that 30 of the biopsies contained micro-papillary DCIS. Follow-up information was only available for 15 of the 30 DCIS patients. In the 15 available, 8 developed invasive breast cancer in the same breast as the DCIS, with an average time to development of 9 years. Similarly, a study conducted by Eusebi et al. investigated 9000 biopsies looking for misdiagnosed cases of DCIS. Out of the 9000 biopsies performed, 80 of them were found to be DCIS. In the 80 cases, 11 developed an invasive cancer over the course of an average of 17.5 years. The results from these misdiagnosis studies can be seen in Table 5.1. These studies suggest that patients with DCIS that were misdiagnosed and who received no further treatment have a risk ranging from 14 to 53% of developing invasive breast cancer 10–15 years later [56]. Taken together, these studies reaffirm the fact that a significantly large subset of DCIS was never destined to become invasive ductal carcinoma.

Autopsy studies provide yet another line of evidence that DCIS does not always progress to invasive disease. The breast tissue of women who died of other causes was studied intensively in a number of studies looking for occult DCIS. The Nielson et al. autopsy study consists of 77 cases, 14 of which were found to have DCIS that the patient was unaware of prior to her death. This incidence rate is significantly higher than unselected screening mammography rates. Gilbert Welch and Robert Black performed a review of seven autopsy studies and found that the average prevalence of DCIS between them all was 8.9%. This is in sharp contrast to screening data which suggests that 1 woman per 1000 per year will be found to have DCIS. The implication is clear.

A more contemporary argument for the natural history of breast cancer comes from a recent large retrospective review of nearly 3000 consecutive cases of DCIS treated with breast conservation. Van Zee et al. reviewed their experience at Memorial Sloan Kettering Cancer Center over a three-decade period. In their patient population, they identified 271 patients with margins of 2 mm or less and another 59 women with documented positive margins. These patients had no further surgery, no radiation therapy, and no endocrine ablative interventions. At 20 years of

Table 5.1 Review of follow-up studies of DCIS initially misdiagnosed as benign lesions

Study	Number of benign biopsies examined	Number of misdiagnosed DCIS [Number for whom follow-up available]	Number subsequently invasive	Age at initial biopsy	Histology	Follow-up period (years)	% invasive (95%CI)[a]
Eusebi et al.	9520 (histological reassessment only on 9446)	80 [80]	11	24–77 years	Comedo and non-comedo	1–14 years	0.14 (0.07, 0.23)
Page et al.	11,760	20 [20]	9	33–74 years	Non-comedo	3–31 years	0.32 (0.15, 0.49)
Rosen et al.[b]	>8000 reported as benign	30 [15]	8	Not reported	Micro-papillary	1–24 years	0.53 (0.28, 0.79)
Collins et al.	1877	13 [13]	6	41–63 years	Not reported	4–18 years	0.46 (0.19, 0.73)

[a]Exact binomial distribution

[b]Same group of patients as Betsill et al. [7] with extended follow-up

Permission applied for: Fong et al. [56]

follow-up, more than 60% of these patients were alive free of invasive breast cancer [57].

5.9   Patient Perception of Risk and Treatment Choice

A study done by Rakovitch et al. [58] found that women with DCIS have the same psychosocial morbidity as women with invasive BC, despite the difference in severity between the two. Additionally, patients also overestimate the benefit of a mastectomy in this clinical setting. Patients do not draw a clear distinction between invasive and in situ disease and this may lead to over-treatment. McCaffery et al. [59] recently published an analysis exploring how different terminology used to describe DCIS has a significant impact on a woman's concern and, eventually, the treatment she selects. The study used the two different phrases to describe the DCIS. The first term used was 'abnormal cells' and the second phrase used was 'pre-invasive breast cancer cells.' If the term 'abnormal cells' is used instead of 'pre-invasive breast cancer cells,' then the patient will be more likely to choose a watchful waiting (active surveillance) approach rather than treat it surgically. These studies have implications for clinicians endeavoring to treat DCIS.

5.10   Role of Radiation in DCIS

The current standard of care in the USA for DCIS treated with breast conservation includes both wide local excision to clear margins and postsurgical radiation therapy. The trial that established that standard was the NSABP B-17 trial [60]. The trial compares lumpectomy alone to lumpectomy with radiation therapy in women with DCIS excised with clear margins. After 10 years, 94.5% of patients remained disease-free after being treated with both lumpectomy and radiation while 83.6% of patients treated with lumpectomy alone remained disease-free, a difference of 10.9%. This difference was both statistically and clinically significant. In the final statement of the published article, the authors stated that they could not identify any subgroup of patients who did not benefit from RT. It is clear that they were not reporting that all groups benefited equally, as 80% of the non-irradiated group remained free of disease at more than 20 years of follow-up. Instead, the authors were acknowledging that the technology was not available to identify a low-risk subgroup whom would not benefit from radiation therapy. At more than 25 years of follow-up, there is no survival advantage in the group who received radiation therapy as part of their breast-conserving approach to DCIS.

Radiation therapy to the breast is associated with a well-characterized list of possible complications. The most common short-term side effects for RT include: axillary discomfort, chest pain, fatigue, lowered white blood cell count, skin burns, itching, pulmonary function impairment, discoloration of the breast, and breast

Table 5.2 Percent increase in rate of major coronary events as a function of the mean dose of radiation to the heart

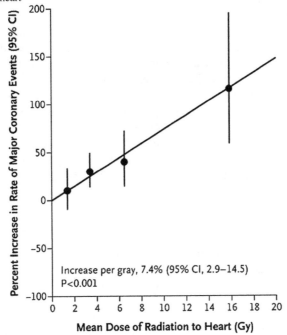

contraction. Two major long-term co-morbidities associated with RT is an increased likelihood of a coronary event and the rare development of a radiation-induced secondary cancer, most commonly angiosarcoma of the breast.

A study done by Darby et al. [61] found that the rate of a coronary event occurring in a patient increased by 7.4% for every Gy administered to the breast (Table 5.2). The study also shows that radiating the left breast caused higher rates of coronary episodes than radiating only the right breast (P = 0.002). Of the 963 women included in the study who suffered a coronary event, 44% of the women experienced the event within 10 years after their BC diagnosis, some even experiencing it as early as 5 years after diagnosis.

Merino et al. [62] demonstrated that, after breast-conserving surgery for early-stage breast cancer patients who are currently treated with a wide range of radiation techniques including whole breast irradiation (WBI), accelerated partial breast irradiation (APBI) using high-dose-rate (HDR) brachytherapy, or 3D-conformal radiotherapy (3D-CRT) all receive some radiation directly to cardiac muscle. The authors compared the mean heart's doses for a left breast irradiated with different breast techniques. Following the model reported by Darby, total cardiac doses were estimated assuming a linear risk increase with the mean dose to the heart of 7.4% per Gy. WBI leads to the highest mean heart dose (2.99 Gy) compared to 3D-CRT APBI (0.51 Gy), multicatheter (1.58 Gy), and balloon HDR (2.17 Gy) for a medially located tumor. This translated into long-term coronary event increases of 22, 3.8, 11.7, and 16%, respectively. The sensitivity analysis showed that the tumor location had almost no effect on the mean heart dose for 3D-CRT APBI and a minimal impact for HDR APBI. In the case of whole breast radiotherapy, large breast size and setup errors lead to sharp increases in the mean heart dose. The total cardiac does reached 10.79 Gy for women with large breast and a setup error of only 1.5 cm. Such a high value could increase the risk of having long-term coronary events by as much as 80%. Comparison among different irradiation techniques demonstrates that 3D-CRT APBI appears to be the safest one with less probability of having cardiovascular events in the future. A sensitivity analysis showed that WBI is the most challenging technique for patients with large breasts or when significant setup errors are unavoidable. In those cases, additional heart shielding techniques are required.

5.11 Tools for Predicting Class in DCIS Treated with Breast Conservation

1. Van Nuys Prognostic Index

The University of Southern California/Van Nuys Prognostic Index (USC/VNPI) is an algorithm that quantifies five measurable prognostic factors known to be important in predicting local recurrence in conservatively treated patients with DCIS. These factors include tumor size, margin width, nuclear grade, age, and the presence or absence of comedonecrosis. The algorithm produces a numerical score that is closely correlated with outcome. A recent publication with considerably more statistical power than the original description allows for subset analysis by individual scores rather than by groups of scores. For example, to achieve a local recurrence rate of less than 20% at 12 years, the USC/VNPI data support excision alone for all patients scoring 4, 5, or 6 and patients who score 7 but have margin widths ≥ 3 mm. Excision plus RT achieves less than 20% local recurrence threshold at 12 years for patients who score 7 and have margins <3 mm, patients who score 8 and have margins ≥ 3 mm, and for patients who score 9 and have margins ≥ 5mm. Mastectomy is recommended for patients who score 8 and have margins <3 mm, who score 9 and have margins <5 mm and for all patients who score 10, 11, or 12 to keep the local recurrence rate less than 20% at 12 years. Silverstein et al. deserve considerable credit for being among the first investigators to report that DCIS behaves as a family of diseases and that any 'one size fits all' approach to therapy will necessarily over-treat a subset of patients. Because of the technical considerations in achieving accurate tumor size and accurate tumor margin size, the USC/VNPI has had limited generalized application. Achieving data that is accurate and reproducible requires subspecialized breast cancer pathology support which most centers do not have [63].

2. MSKCC Nomogram

Van Zee et al. at Memorial Sloan Kettering Cancer Center sought to individualize the estimation of ipsilateral breast tumor recurrence (IBTR) in patients treated conservatively for DCIS by developing a nomogram based upon a multivariate Cox proportional hazards model. From 1991 to 2006, 1868 consecutive patients treated with breast conservation for DCIS were identified. The model was constructed using the 1681 in which data were complete. Ten clinical, pathologic, and treatment variables were built into a nomogram estimating probability of IBTR at 5 and 10 years after BCS. The model was validated for discrimination and calibration using bootstrap resampling.

The DCIS nomogram for prediction of 5- and 10-year IBTR probabilities demonstrated reasonable calibration and discrimination, with a concordance index of 0.704 (bootstrap corrected, 0.688) and a concordance probability estimate of 0.686. This concordance probability has been interpreted in a variety of ways by other groups attempting to validate the nomogram. The factors with the greatest influence on risk of IBTR in the model included adjuvant RT or endocrine therapy, age, margin status, number of excisions, and treatment time period. The authors have concluded that the tool is an useful adjunct in the decision-making process regarding the treatment of DCIS. They further claim that the nomogram has been 'validated' by at least four groups independently [64]. It is correct that the four outside groups all came to similar conclusions regarding the C-index score (all ranged from 6.1 to 6.9) with a score of 1 being perfect concordance and a score of 0.5 being no concordance whatsoever. Most statistical texts report C-Index scores of 0.6–0.7 as fair to poor.

One of the groups that attempted to validate the utility of the MSKCC nomogram was the group at MD Anderson Cancer Center [65]. The aim of their study was to evaluate the nomogram in their patient population. They retrospectively identified 794 patients with a diagnosis of DCIS who had undergone local excision from 1990 to 2007 at the MD Anderson Cancer Center (MDACC). Clinicopathologic factors and the performance of the Memorial Sloan Kettering Cancer Center nomogram for prediction of IBTR were assessed for 734 patients who had complete data. In their analysis, there was a marked difference with respect to tumor grade, prevalence of necrosis, initial presentation, final margins, and receipt of endocrine therapy between the MSKCC and MDAC cohorts. The biggest difference was that more patients received radiation in the MDACC cohort (75% at MDACC vs. 49% at MSKCC; $P < 0.001$). Follow-up time in the MDACC cohort was longer than in the MSKCC cohort (median 7.1 years vs. 5.6 years), and the recurrence rate was lower in the MDACC cohort (7.9% vs. 11%). The median five-year probability of recurrence was 5%, and the median ten-year probability of recurrence was 7%. The authors concluded that the MSKCC nomogram for prediction of five- and 1ten-year IBTR probabilities demonstrated imperfect calibration and discrimination, with a concordance index of 0.63. They concluded that predicting recurrence on the basis of clinical parameters alone is limited. The nomogram provided a valuable tool in an era before genomic profiling was available and the contribution of Van Zee and her colleagues should be acknowledged.

3. Genomic Profiling and the Era of Precision Medicine

The 8th Revision of the American Joint Commission on Cancer Staging system, set to become effective on January 1, 2018, will provide both anatomic staging and prognostic staging for breast cancer. The only platform with level 1 evidence supporting prognostic and predictive information in the new system is the 21 gene assay (Oncotype DX). This assay provides personalized information for tailoring treatment based on the biology of a patient's individual disease. The test is supported by multiple rigorous clinical validation studies confirming the test's ability to predict the likelihood of chemotherapy benefit as well as the chance of cancer recurrence in early-stage breast cancer. The test is intended for use in all newly diagnosed patients with early-stage (stage I, II, or IIIa) breast cancer who have node-negative or node-positive (1–3), estrogen receptor-positive (ER+), HER2-negative disease. As the only test proven to predict chemotherapy benefit, the 21 gene assay test is included in all major cancer guidelines worldwide and now considered as standard of care for women with early-stage breast cancer with unprecedented prospective patient outcomes in more than 50,000 patients from four large, independently run, international studies. These positive results from the SEER Registry, TAILORx, Clalit and West German Group's Plan B studies demonstrate that the 21 gene assay accurately predicts patient outcomes—including risk of recurrence and breast cancer survival. The studies showed that 99% of those with low 21 gene assay scores who were primarily treated using hormonal therapy alone, without chemotherapy, were cancer free after 5 years [66].

Researchers investigating DCIS selected a subset of 12 genes from the 21 gene assay and sought to create and validate an assay that would predict the risk of local recurrence in non-radiated patients at ten years of follow-up. The first study to be reported represented an analysis of archival DCIS from the ECOG5194 trial. The platform was created, validated, and eventually used to investigate the DCIS tissue in the tumor bank from ECOG5194. This type of research, labeled as retrospective/prospective, provides critical information about innate tumor genomics and can predict recurrence class. Solin et al. reported the results of their analysis of patients in the ECOG 5194 study and found that the score does, in fact, quantify the risk of DCIS. The results of the analysis were as follows, 10.6, 26.7, and 25.9% were the 10-year rates of developing IBE for low-, intermediate-, and high-risk groups, respectively, (p = 0.006) and 3.7, 12.3, and 19.2% are the 10-year rates of developing invasive IBE for low-, intermediate-, and high-risk groups, respectively, (p = 0.003). The study concluded that the risk of developing IBE was significantly lower for the 70% of patients with a low DCIS score as compared to the 30% of patients with a high DCIS score [67, 68].

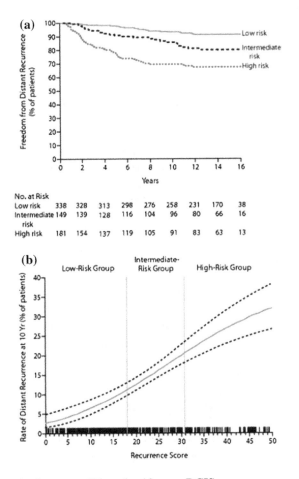

A second study done to validate the 12 gene DCIS recurrence score capitalized on archival tumor tissue from a large tumor bank in Ontario Province, Canada. The objective was to confirm the results of the ECOG 5194 study in a larger population-based cohort of individuals with DCIS treated with BCS alone from 1994 to 2003. The Cox model was used to determine the relationship between independent covariates, the disease-free survival [hazard ratio (HR)/50 Cp units (U)] and local recurrence (LR). Tumor blocks were collected for 828 patients.

The final evaluable population included 718 cases, of whom 571 had negative margins. The median follow-up was 9.6 years over which time 100 cases developed LR following BCS alone (DCIS, N = 44; invasive, N = 57). In the primary pre-specified analysis, the disease-free survival was associated with any LR (DCIS or invasive) in ER+ patients (HR 2.26; P < 0.001) and in all patients regardless of ER status (HR 2.15; P < 0.001). The 12 gene assay (DCIS score) provided independent information on LR risk beyond clinical and pathologic variables including size, age, grade, necrosis, multifocality, and subtype (adjusted HR 1.68; P = 0.02).

DCIS was associated with invasive LR (HR 1.78; P = 0.04) and DCIS LR (HR 2.43; P = 0.005).

The authors concluded that the 12 gene DCIS score assay independently predicts and quantifies individualized recurrence risk in a population of patients with pure DCIS treated by BCS alone. Finally, the Ontario Province dataset and outcomes matched the ECOG study outcome very closely despite the fact that it included a population-based group of tumor samples, different surgeons, different treatment approaches in a different country [69].

In an attempt to further validate the 12 gene assay for DCIS, thirteen sites across the USA enrolled patients from March 2014 through August 2015 with pure DCIS undergoing breast conservation therapy. Prospectively collected data included clinic–pathologic factors, physician estimates of local recurrence risk, DCIS score results, and pre-/post-assay radiotherapy recommendations for each patient made by a surgeon and a radiation oncologist.

Patients completed pre- and post-assay decisional conflict scale and state-trait anxiety inventory instruments. The analysis cohort included 127 patients: median age 60 years. Eighty percent were postmenopausal. The median tumor size was 8 mm (39% $\leq$ 5 mm), 70% grade 1/2, 88% estrogen receptor-positive, 75% progesterone receptor-positive, 54% with comedo necrosis, and 18% were multifocal. Similar to the results of the ECOG and Ontario Province data, 66% of patients had low DCIS score results; 20% had intermediate DCIS score results, and 14% had high DCIS score results; the median result was 21 (range 0–84).

Pre-assay, surgeons, and radiation oncologists recommended radiotherapy for 70.9 and 72.4% of patients, respectively. Post-assay, 26.4% of overall recommendations changed, including 30.7 and 22.0% of recommendations by surgeons and radiation oncologists, respectively. Among patients with confirmed completed questionnaires (n = 32), decision conflict (p = 0.004) and state anxiety (p = 0.042) decreased significantly from pre- to post-assay. The authors concluded that the individualized risk estimates from the DCIS score assay provided valuable information to physicians and patients. Post-assay, in response to DCIS score results, surgeons changed treatment recommendations more often than radiation oncologists [70].

5.12 Conclusion

DCIS has been poorly understood since its original description nearly three quarters of a century ago. Unjustified comparisons to invasive ductal carcinoma, partially misinterpreted clinical trials and public misconceptions about the disease have aligned in support of over-treatment in some women with DCIS. Ductal carcinoma in situ is not an obligate precursor to invasive ductal carcinoma. The majority of cases of DCIS were either unlikely to progress to invasive cancer or were going to invade at a very slow pace. There are still many unanswered questions regarding DCIS. In the majority of patients, DCIS is not actually a disease but rather a pathologic finding associated with an increased risk of developing invasive carcinoma. It is reasonable to assume, in the future, that DCIS found on core biopsy may be subjected to gene expression profiling and low-risk lesions may not be removed. Without question, genomic profiling holds the highest promise for accurate class prediction in the condition and is the best chance to achieve a reasonable reconciliation of a means to an end in treating DCIS.

References

1. Marshall BJ (1983) Unidentified curved bacillus on gastric epithelium in active chronic gastritis. Lancet 1(8336):1273–1275. doi:10.1016/S0140-6736(83)92719-8. PMID 6134060
2. Marshall BJ, Warren JR (1984) Unidentified curved bacilli in the stomach patients with gastritis and peptic ulceration. Lancet 1(8390):1311–1315. doi:10.1016/S0140-6736(84)91816-6. PMID 6145023
3. Sørum R1, Hofvind S, Skaane P, Haldorsen T (2010) Trends in incidence of ductal carcinoma in situ: the effect of a population-based screening programme. 19(6):499–505. doi: 10.1016/j.breast.2010.05.014. Epub 2010 June 17
4. Jorgensen KJ, Gotzsche PC (2009) Overdiagnosis in publicly organised mammography screening programmes: systematic review of incidence trends. BMJ 339:B2587
5. Kumar AS, Bhatia V, Henderson IC (2005) Overdiagnosis and overtreatment of breast cancer: Rates of ductal carcinoma in situ: a US perspective. Breast Cancer Research 7(6):271–275
6. Page DL, Dupont WD, Rogers LW, Landenberger M (1982) Intraductal carcinoma of the breast: follow-up after biopsy only. Cancer 49:751–758
7. Betsill WL, Rosen PP, Lieberman PH, Robbins GF (1978) Intraductal carcinoma: long-term follow-up after treatment by biopsy alone. JAMA 239:1863–1867
8. Rosen P, Snyder RE, Foote FW, Wallace T (1970) Detection of occult carcinoma in the apparently benign breast biopsy through speci- men radiography. Cancer 26:944–952
9. Eusebi V, Feudale E, Foschini MP, Micheli A, Conti A, Riva C, Di Palma S, Rilke F (1994) Long-term follow-up of in situ carcinoma of the breast. Semin Diagn Pathol 11:223–235
10. Erbas B, Provenzano E, Armes J et al (2006) Breast Cancer Res Treat 97:135. doi:10.1007/s10549-005-9101-z
11. Nielsen M, Jensen J, Andersen J (1984) Precancerous and cancerous breast lesions during lifetime and at autopsy. A study of 83 women. Cancer 54:612–615. doi:10.1002/1097-0142(1984)54:4<612:AID-CNCR2820540403>3.0.CO;2-B
12. Welch HG, Black WC (1997) Using autopsy series to estimate the disease "reservoir" for ductal carcinoma in situ of the breast: how much more breast cancer can we find? Ann Intern Med. 127:1023–1028. doi:10.7326/0003-4819-127-11-199712010-0001
13. Van Zee KJ, Subhedar P, Olcese C et al (2015) Relationship between margin width and recurrence of ductal carcinoma in situ: analysis of 2996 women treated with breast conserving surgery for 30 years. Ann Surg 262(4):623–631
14. Collins LC, Tamimi RM, Baer HJ et al (2005) Outcome of patients with ductal carcinoma in situ untreated after diagnostic biopsy: results from the Nurses' Health Study. Cancer 103:1778–1784
15. Birkett J (1850) e diseases of the breast and eir treatment. Longman, London
16. Cornil AV (1865) Contributions a l'histoire du developement histologique des tumeurs epithelial. J Anat Physiol 2:266–276
17. Ribbert H (1911) Das Karzinom des Menschen. F. Cohen, Bonn
18. Ewing J (1919) Neoplastic diseases. Saunders, Philadelphia
19. Masson P (1923) Traite de Pathologie Medicale et de erapeutique Appliquee. A. Maloine, Paris

20. Cheatle GL, Cutler M (1931) Tumours of the breast. Lippincott, Philadelphia
21. Broders AC (1932) Carcinoma in situ contrasted with benign penetrating epithelium. JAMA 99:1670–1674
22. Foote FW, Stewart FW (1932) Lobular carcinoma in situ. A rare form of mammary cance. Am J Path 17:491–496
23. Stewart FW (1950) Tumors of the Breast. Armed Forces Institute of Pathology, Washington, DC
24. Francis A, Thomas J, Fallowfield L et al (2015) Addressing overtreatment of screen detected DCIS; the LORIS trial. Eur J Cancer 51:2296–2303
25. Ernster VL, Barclay J (1997) Increases in ductal carcinoma in situ (DCIS) of the breast in relation to mammography: a dilemma. J Natl Cancer Inst Monogr 22:151–156
26. Wellings SR, Jensen HM (1973) On the origin and progression of ductal carcinoma in the human breast. J Natl Cancer Inst 50:1111–1118
27. Page DL, Dupont WD, Rogers LW et al (1995) Continued local recurrence of carcinoma 15–25 years after a diagnosis of low grade ductal carcinoma in situ of the breast treated only by biopsy. Cancer 76:1197–1200
28. Dupont WD, Page DL (1985) Risk factors for breast cancer in women with proliferative breast disease. N Engl J Med 312:146–151
29. Tavassoli FA (1998) Ductal carcinoma in situ: introduction of the concept of ductal intraepithelial neoplasia. Mod Pathol 11:140–154
30. McCaffery K, Nickel B, Moynihan R et al (2015) How different terminology for ductal carcinoma in situ impacts women's concern and treatment preferences: a randomised comparison within a national community survey. BMJ Open 5:e008094
31. Bartlett JM, Nofech-Moses S, Rakovitch E (2014) Ductal carcinoma in situ of the breast: can biomarkers improve current management? Clin Chem 60:60–67
32. Thompson A, Brennan K, Cox A et al (2008) Evaluation of the current knowledge limitations in breast cancer research: a gap analysis. Breast Cancer Res 10:R26
33. Leonard GD, Swain SM (2004) Ductal carcinoma in situ, complexities and challenges. J Natl Cancer Inst 96:906–920
34. Aubele M, Mattis A, Zitzelsberger H et al (1999) Intratumoral heterogeneity in breast carcinoma revealed by laser-microdissection and comparative genomic hybridization. Cancer Genet Cytogenet 110:94–102
35. Aubele M, Cummings M, Walsch A et al (2000) Heterogeneous chromosomal aberrations in intraductal breast lesions adjacent to invasive carcinoma. Anal Cell Pathol 20:17–24
36. Aubele M, Mattis A, Zitzelsberger H et al (2000) Extensive ductal carcinoma in situ with small foci of invasive ductal carcinoma: evidence of genetic resemblance by CGH. Int J Cancer 85:82–86
37. Foschini MP, Morandi L, Leonardi E et al (2013) Genetic clonal mapping of in situ and invasive ductal carcinoma indicates the field cancerization phenomenon in the breast. Hum Pathol 44:1310–1319
38. Luzzi V, Holtschlag V, Watson MA (2001) Expression profiling of ductal carcinoma in situ by laser capture microdissection and high-density oligonucleotide arrays. Am J Pathol 158:2005–2010
39. Reis-Filho JS, Lakhani SR (2003) The diagnosis and management of pre-invasive breast disease: genetic alterations in pre-invasive lesions. Breast Cancer Res 5:313–319
40. Werner M, Mattis A, Aubele M et al (1999) 20q13.2 amplification in intraductal hyperplasia adjacent to in situ and invasive ductal carcinoma of the breast. Virchows Arch 435:469–472
41. Westbury CB, Reis-Filho JS, Dexter T et al (2009) Genome-wide transcriptomic profiling of microdissected human breast tissue reveals differential expression of KIT (c-Kit, CD117) and oestrogen receptor-alpha (ERalpha) in response to therapeutic radiation. J Pathol 219:131–140

42. Ghazani AA, Arneson N, Warren K et al (2007) Genomic alterations in sporadic synchronous primary breast cancer using array and metaphase comparative genomic hybridization. Neoplasia 9:511–520

43. Hernandez L, Wilkerson PM, Lambros MB et al (2012) Genomic and mutational profiling of ductal carcinomas in situ and matched adjacent invasive breast cancers reveals intra-tumour genetic heterogeneity and clonal selection. J Pathol 227:42–52

44. Kim SY, Jung SH, Kim MS et al (2015) Genomic differences between pure ductal carcinoma in situ and synchronous ductal carcinoma in situ with invasive breast cancer. Oncotarget 6:7597–7607

45. Kroigard AB, Larsen MJ, Laenkholm AV et al (2015) Clonal expansion and linear genome evolution through breast cancer progression from pre-invasive stages to asynchronous metastasis. Oncotarget 6:5634–5649

46. Koboldt DC, Steinberg KM, Larson DE et al (2013) The next-generation sequencing revolution and its impact on genomics. Cell 155:27–38

47. Newburger DE, Kashef-Haghighi D, Weng Z et al (2013) Genome evolution during progression to breast cancer. Genome Res 23:1097–1108

48. Yates LR, Gerstung M, Knappskog S et al (2015) Subclonal diversification of primary breast cancer revealed by multiregion sequencing. Nature Med 21:751–759

49. Fujii H, Szumel R, Marsh C et al (1996) Genetic progression, histological grade, and allelic loss in ductal carcinoma in situ of the breast. Cancer Res 56:5260–5265

50. Buerger H, Mommers EC, Littmann R et al (2001) Ductal invasive G2 and G3 carcinomas of the breast are the end stages of at least two different lines of genetic evolution. J Pathol 194:165–170

51. Roylance R, Gorman P, Harris W et al (1999) Comparative genomic hybridization of breast tumors stratified by histological grade reveals new insights into the biological progression of breast cancer. Cancer Res 59:1433–1436

52. Simpson PT, Gale T, Reis-Filho JS et al (2005) Columnar cell lesions of the breast: the missing link in breast cancer progression? A morphological and molecular analysis. Am J Surg Pathol 29:734–746

53. Shackney SE, Silverman JF (2003) Molecular evolutionary patterns in breast cancer. Adv Anat Pathol 10:278–290

54. Buerger H, Otterbach F, Simon R et al (1999) Comparative genomic hybridization of ductal carcinoma in situ of the breast—evidence of multiple genetic pathways. J Pathol 187:396–402

55. Johnson CE, Gorringe KL, Thompson ER et al (2012) Identification of copy number alterations associated with the progression of DCIS to invasive ductal carcinoma. Breast Cancer Res Treat 133:889–898

56. Fong J, Kurniawan ED, Rose AK et al (2011) Ann Surg Oncol 18:3778. doi:10.1245/s10434-011-1748-6

57. Van Zee KJ, Subhedar P, Olcese C et al (2015) Relationship between margin width and recurrence of ductal carcinoma in situ: analysis of 2996 women treated with breast conserving surgery for 30 years. Ann Surg 262(4):623–631

58. Rakovitch E, Nofech-Mozes S, Hanna W, Baehner FL, Saskin R, Butler SM, Paszat L (2015) A population-based validation study of the DCIS score predicting recurrence risk in individuals treated by breast-conserving surgery alone. Breast Cancer Res Treat 152(2):389–398

59. McCaffery K, Nickel B, Moynihan R, Hersch J, Teixeira-Pinto A, Irwig L, Barratt A (2015) How different terminology for ductal carcinoma in situ impacts women's concern and treatment preferences: a randomised comparison within a national community survey. BMJ Open 5(11):e008094. doi:10.1136/bmjopen-2015-008094

60. Wapnir IL, Dignam JJ, Fisher B, Mamounas EP, Anderson SJ, Julian TB, Land SR, Margolese RG, Swain SM, Costantino JP, Wolmark N (2011) Long-term outcomes of invasive ipsilateral breast tumor recurrences after lumpectomy in NSABP B-17 and B-24

randomized clinical trials for DCIS. J Natl Cancer Inst 103(6): 478–488. doi:10.1093/jnci/djr027. Epub 2011 Mar 11

61. Darby SC, Ewertz M, McGale P, Bennet AM, Blom-Goldman U, Dorthe Brønnum RN, Correa C, Cutter D, Gagliardi G, Gigante B, Jensen M-J, Nibset A, Nibset A, Richard Peto FRS, Kazem Rahimi DM, Taylor C, Hall P (2013) N Engl J Med 368(11):987–998. doi:10.1056/NEJMoa1209825

62. Merino Lara TR, Fleury E, Mashouf S, Helou J, McCann C, Ruschin M, Kim A, Makhani N, Ravi A, Pignol JP (2014) Measurement of mean cardiac dose for various breast irradiation techniques and corresponding risk of major cardiovascular event. Front Oncol 22(4):284. doi:10.3389/fonc.2014.00284

63. Silverstein MJ, Lagios MD (2010) Choosing treatment for patients with ductal carcinoma in situ: fine tuning the University of Southern California/Van Nuys Prognostic Index. J Natl Cancer Inst Monogr 2010(41):193–196. doi:10.1093/jncimonographs/lgq040

64. Rudloff U, Jacks LM, Goldberg JI, Wynveen CA, Brogi E, Patil S, Van Zee KJ (2010) Nomogram for predicting the risk of local recurrence after breast-conserving surgery for ductal carcinoma in situ. J Clin Oncol 28(23):3762–3769. doi:10.1200/JCO.2009.26.8847. Epub 2010 July 12

65. Yi M, Meric-Bernstam F, Kuerer HM, Mittendorf EA, Bedrosian I, Lucci A, Hwang RF, Crow JR, Luo S, Hunt KK (2012) Evaluation of a breast cancer nomogram for predicting risk of ipsilateral breast tumor recurrences in patients with ductal carcinoma in situ after local excision. Clin Oncol 30(6):600–607. doi:10.1200/JCO.2011.36.4976. Epub 2012 Jan 17

66. Sparano JA, Gray RJ, Makower DF, Pritchard KI, Albain KS, Hayes DF, Geyer CE Jr, Dees EC, Perez EA, Olson JA Jr, Zujewski J, Lively T, Badve SS, Saphner TJ, Wagner LI, Whelan TJ, Ellis MJ, Paik S, Wood WC, Ravdin P, Keane MM, Gomez Moreno HL, Reddy PS, Goggins TF, Mayer IA, Brufsky AM, Toppmeyer DL, Kaklamani VG, Atkins JN, Berenberg JL, Sledge GW (2015) Prospective Validation of a 21-gene expression assay in breast cancer. N Eng J Med 373(21):2005–2014. doi:10.1056/NEJMoa1510764. Epub 2015 Sept 27

67. Darby SC, Ewertz M, McGale P, Bennet AM, Blom-Goldman U, Brønnum D, Correa C, Cutter D, Gagliardi G, Gigante B, Jensen MB, Nisbet A, Peto R, Rahimi K, Taylor C, Hall P (2013) Risk of ischemic heart disease in women after radiotherapy for breast cancer. N Engl J Med 368:987–998 March 14, 2013. DOI: 10.1056/NEJMoa1209825

68. Solin LJ, Gray R, Hughes LL et al (2015) Surgical excision without radiation for ductal carcinoma in situ of the breast: 12-year results from the ECOG-ACRIN E5194 study. J Clin Oncol 33:3938–3944

69. Rakovitch E, Nofech-Mozes S, Hanna W et al (2015) A population-based validation study of the DCIS Score predicting recurrence risk in individuals treated by breast-conserving surgery alone. Breast Cancer Res Treat 152(2):389–398. doi:10.1007/s10549-015-3464-6

70. Manders JB1, Kuerer HM2, Smith BD2, McCluskey C3, Farrar WB4, Frazier TG5, Li L5, Leonard CE6, Carter DL6, Chawla S7, Medeiros LE7, Guenther JM8, Castellini LE8, Buchholz DJ9, Mamounas EP9, Wapnir IL10, Horst KC10, Chagpar A11, Evans SB11, Riker AI12,13, Vali FS12, Solin LJ14, Jablon L14, Recht A15, Sharma R15, Lu R16, Sing AP16, Hwang ES17, White J4 (2017) Study investigators and study participants. Clinical utility of the 12-gene DCIS score assay: impact on radiotherapy recommendations for patients with ductal carcinoma in situ. Ann Surg Oncol 24(3):660–668. doi:10.1245/s10434-016-5583-7. Epub 2016 Oct 4

Readdressing the Role of Surgery of the Primary Tumor in de Novo Stage IV Breast Cancer

6

Seema Ahsan Khan and Elizabeth S. M. DesJardin

Contents

S. A. Khan (✉)
Robert H. Lurie Comprehensive Cancer Center, 301 East Superior Street,
Room 4-111, Chicago, IL 60611, USA
e-mail: s-khan2@northwestern.edu

E. S. M. DesJardin
Northwestern McGaw Medical Center, 250 East Superior, Suite 4-420,
Chicago, IL 60611, USA
e-mail: elizabeth.jardin@northwestern.edu

© Springer International Publishing AG 2018
W. J. Gradishar (ed.), *Optimizing Breast Cancer Management*, Cancer Treatment
and Research 173, https://doi.org/10.1007/978-3-319-70197-4_6

Abstract

The impressive advances in breast cancer treatment observed in recent years also apply to the metastatic setting, where a subset of patients with favorable metastatic disease enjoy long-term survival with systemic therapy. In patients with distant disease, the primary tumor in the breast has not classically been though to merit specific locoregional therapy. However, about 6% of Stage IV patients in the USA and up to 20% in limited resource environments present with synchronous distant metastases at the time of initial diagnosis. For this group, who have an intact primary tumor, retrospective studies suggest that local therapy for the primary site may be beneficial. However, these retrospective analyses are biased in that women receiving local therapy to the primary site were younger and had biologically favorable tumors and lower volume metastatic disease. Two completed randomized clinical trials have shown conflicting results, and others are ongoing. In this chapter, we discuss the results of these studies through the present day and summarize their conclusions and their implications for clinical management.

Keywords

Stage IV breast cancer · Local therapy · Locoregional therapy
Surgery · Metastatic breast cancer · Survival

6.1   Introduction

Stage IV breast cancer has begun to resemble a chronic disease in some patients thanks to advances in diagnostic technology and a myriad of systemic therapy options. A subset of patients with limited metastatic disease can realize long-term survival when treated with multimodality therapy [1, 2]. In some women with Stage IV breast cancer, metastases may be the presenting symptom, or may be diagnosed at the same time as the primary tumor. This group of patients with de novo Stage IV disease makes up about 6% of new breast cancer diagnoses in the USA and Western Europe [3]. Here too, temporal trends show improvements in survival. In a 2004 study from France which examined 724 patients with de novo metastatic breast cancer, a 27% of patients survived for 3 years if diagnosed from 1987 to 1993, whereas 44% survived for 3 years if diagnosed between 1994 and 2000 [4]. A more recent American study based on data from the Surveillance, Epidemiology and End Results (SEER) registries of the National Cancer Institute shows similar trends [5]. With the time period 1988–1991 as reference, hazard ratios improved steadily to 2007–2001, when they were observed to be 0.81 (95% CI 0.74, 0.88). This improvement is likely multifactorial, partly explained by lead-time bias from improved diagnostic imaging and partly by a true improvement in survival related to better therapy.

The mainstay of treatment for metastatic breast cancer is systemic therapy including a variety of chemotherapeutic agents as well as endocrine and targeted therapies customized to each patient and their tumor features [6]. With this combination of lead-time bias and increasingly more effective therapy, many patients with de novo metastatic disease are now living with an intact primary tumor for years. Traditionally, the primary site has been managed with systemic therapy, in the expectation that local and systemic responses occur in parallel and the primary will remain in check using medical therapy. The notion that treatment of the primary tumor would aid survival has gained currency in recent years [7]. Although local progression of the tumor is an obvious risk to quality of life in some patients, objective data are needed to document both the local control benefits of local therapy and any putative effects on survival.

6.2 Arguments for Local Therapy to the Primary Tumor

For patients, resection of the primary is intuitively appealing and gives a sense of concrete progress toward decreased volume of disease. From a more objective standpoint, physicians and patients alike are motivated to avoid the cosmetic and quality of life issues that arise with advanced local disease, and all are interested in any survival advantage that may be offered by primary tumor resection in this Stage IV setting. Examination of other organ system malignancies provides some insight into this question. Metastatic ovarian, gastric, colorectal, and renal cell carcinoma all shows a survival benefit from resection of the primary tumor in retrospective studies [8–11], with renal cell carcinoma being the only disease site where this has been tested in a randomized trial [12, 13]. For Stage IV ovarian cancer, surgical debulking is now standard of care [14] and it is believed that the systemic therapy in these cases is able to penetrate this lower volume of disease more effectively.

Investigations of cancer stem cells (CSCs) and circulating tumor cells (CTCs) provide further conceptual support for resection of the primary tumor. It is thought that these cells can facilitate signaling between the metastatic sites and the primary tumor [15]. CSCs derived from the primary tumor may be more efficient in seeding metastatic colonies that are competent to grow at distant sites, thus propagating the burden of disease [16, 17]. The rationale for primary tumor resection in this case therefore would be to remove a major source of metastatically competent circulating tumor cells, anticipating a corresponding decrease in new sites of metastasis, and prolonged survival.

There is also some evidence suggesting an immunity-related benefit from local treatment of the primary. Resection of the primary in a mouse model of Stage IV breast cancer, for example, re-established the immunocompetence of the host [18]. Other laboratory models have cautioned that removal of the primary site disease may have the opposite effect. One study examined the interaction of two equivalent sites of disease by creating two tumor foci by inoculation with tumor cells; one focus was then resected, and growth was seen in the second site [19]. A similar result was seen when a model with a xenografted tumor was resected and the metastatic lesions showed increased growth [20]. One group showed release of angiogenesis inhibitors by the intact primary tumor in their animal model, which suggests a possible explanation for suppression of metastatic growth by the primary [21]. However, this possible metastatic-suppression effect of the primary tumor has not been observed in humans.

6.3 Review of Retrospective Studies on Resection of Primary Tumor

To date, approximately twenty retrospective studies have examined overall survival outcomes related to primary site local therapy in the setting of Stage IV breast cancer. Overall 27,000 patients were included in multi-institutional and population database research and 14,443 of those had surgery [5, 22–26]. Another 4000 patients were included in thirteen single academic institution analyses from Europe, Asia, and the USA with 1670 of those undergoing surgery [27–40]. Petrelli and Barni utilized fifteen of these retrospective studies in a meta-analysis looking at primary site local therapy (mainly tumor resection) and survival and found a protective association between the two with a hazard ratio of 0.69 ($p < 0.00001$) (Fig. 6.1 Petrelli and Barni). Notably, when examined in conjunction with features including margin status, site of metastases, tumor burden, hormone receptor and HER2 status, age, and type of surgery, the survival advantage seems to be independent (36). Axillary management was more difficult to evaluate in retrospective analyses and is not always detailed well in all these studies.

Study or Subgroup	log[Hazard Ratio]	SE	Weight	Hazard Ratio IV, Random, 95% CI	Year
Khan 2002 R1	-0.286	0.028	10.1%	0.75 [0.71, 0.79]	2002
Khan 2002 R0	-0.491	0.027	10.1%	0.61 [0.58, 0.65]	2002
Rapiti 2006 R0	-0.511	0.261	2.8%	0.60 [0.36, 1.00]	2006
Rapiti 2006 R1	0.262	0.246	3.1%	1.30 [0.80, 2.10]	2006
Babiera 2006	-0.693	0.443	1.2%	0.50 [0.21, 1.19]	2006
Fields 2007	-0.635	0.119	6.7%	0.53 [0.42, 0.67]	2007
Gnerlich 2007	-0.478	0.032	10.0%	0.62 [0.58, 0.66]	2007
Blanchard 2008	-0.342	0.125	6.4%	0.71 [0.56, 0.91]	2008
Hazard 2008	-0.226	0.354	1.8%	0.80 [0.40, 1.60]	2008
Ruiterkamp 2009	-0.478	0.102	7.4%	0.62 [0.51, 0.76]	2009
Bafford 2009	-0.75	0.25	3.0%	0.47 [0.29, 0.77]	2009
Shien 2009	-0.117	0.06	9.1%	0.89 [0.79, 1.00]	2009
Neuman 2010	-0.342	0.217	3.7%	0.71 [0.46, 1.09]	2010
Perez-Fidalgo 2011	-0.654	0.202	4.0%	0.52 [0.35, 0.77]	2011
Dominici 2011	-0.062	0.057	9.2%	0.94 [0.84, 1.05]	2011
Booh Pathy 2011	-0.545	0.093	7.8%	0.58 [0.48, 0.70]	2011
Rashaan 2012	-0.105	0.216	3.7%	0.90 [0.59, 1.37]	2012
Total (95% CI)			100.0%	0.69 [0.63, 0.77]	

Heterogeneity: Tau² = 0.03; Chi² = 110.08, df = 16 (P < 0.00001); I² = 85%
Test for overall effect: Z = 7.15 (P < 0.00001)

0.2   0.5   1   2   5
Favours surgery   Favours no surgery

Fig. 6.1 Pooled analysis of hazard ratios for overall mortality for primary tumor local therapy in patients with stage IV breast cancer

Hartmann et al. performed a meta-analysis comprising six retrospective studies [23, 27, 29, 33, 41, 42] that did include documentation on surgery of the axilla. In this report, 42% of included patients underwent surgery with 69% (527 patients) of these undergoing axillary surgery as well [43]. However, the relationship of axillary surgery to survival in this setting remains unclear as only a few of these studies examined this specifically and no survival benefit was seen from axillary surgery [23, 44].

Locoregional radiotherapy (RT) effect on survival when it is used in addition to surgery is difficult to determine as it is not clearly described in many studies. However, the use of primary radiotherapy has been addressed in at least two studies. A group of 581 patients with synchronous metastasis at the time of their breast cancer diagnosis was reported by Le Scodan et al. [37]. Of these, 320 received locoregional therapy (LRT) and 261 received no LRT. In the LRT group, 249 patients received RT only, 41 received surgery followed by RT, and 30 received surgery alone. Overall, the patients who received RT alone showed a significant survival advantage compared to those who did not (HR 0.7). Another study from British Columbia, with accrual from 1996 to 2005, included 733 patients with metastatic disease and examined outcomes between those treated with LRT of the primary tumor ($n = 378$) versus no LRT ($n = 355$). The five-year overall survival (OS) for these groups was 22% and 14%, respectively ($p < 0.001$). The LRT in this study consisted of surgery only in 67%, RT only for 22%, and both surgery and RT in 11%. The five-year OS for each of these three groups was higher than for no LRT, but the small group with both surgery and RT together showed the highest OS at 32.5% [38]. These studies suggest primary RT may be equivalent to primary surgery when used in patients with metastatic disease, but the fraction of women receiving both surgery and RT to the primary site was too small to allow any conclusions. In these, as in other studies, women with smaller tumors, patients with lower metastatic burden, and hormone receptor-positive disease fared better.

Avoiding symptomatic local disease is another potential advantage of surgical treatment of the primary though retrospective data examining this question are scant. A single-institution study of 111 patients with either de novo metastatic breast cancer or those with distant metastases diagnosed postoperatively examined chest wall outcomes along with survival [42]. Early surgical management of the primary site decreased symptomatic chest wall progression by 86% compared to delayed or no surgical management. Additionally, patients had better survival outcomes (hazard ratio 0.42, $p < 0.002$) if they had sustained chest wall control as opposed to those with uncontrolled chest wall disease. Data from British Columbia are similar: Locoregional progression-free survival was 72% in those receiving any form of locoregional therapy (LRT) than in those who did not (72 vs. 46%, $p < 0.001$) [38].

6.4 Bias in Retrospective Studies

While local therapy seems to contribute favorably to survival in the above studies, these results must be considered carefully in the context of potential bias. Retrospectives studies do not allow analysis of the factors that drive the decisions of physicians and patients. Although known sources of bias can be adjusted for in logistic regression models, some residual confounding cannot be excluded. In addition, unrecognized sources of bias, or those that are difficult to quantify retrospectively, are not possible to correct. Patients who had superior access to care (38, 27) and more favorable characteristics including younger age, fewer comorbidities, non-visceral disease, and smaller tumors were also more likely to have undergone surgery (40, 33, 34). Cases where the diagnosis of Stage IV disease is made after surgery also add bias. For example, some patients initially appear to have Stage I or II disease but are unexpectedly found to have many positive lymph nodes on their surgical pathology. When they subsequently undergo metastatic workup, patients found to have metastases in this scenario will typically have a lower burden of metastatic disease than their counterparts who were found to be Stage IV from the start (40, 41, 26, 44). Registry data are especially susceptible to this type of bias because the stage recorded in the registry is usually months after diagnosis and initial treatment, at which point distant metastasis has typically been found. It is impossible to determine exactly in what way and how significantly these biases effect the outcome data in these studies, thus emphasizing the importance of randomized controlled trials, which will be examined next.

6.5 Randomized Trials

The retrospective data described above led to the initiation of six randomized trials to test the hypothesis that primary site local therapy (PSLT) confers a survival benefit to patients with distant metastases. A randomized trial conducted at Tata Memorial Hospital in Mumbai, India, has reported final results [45]. A Phase III trial performed in the Turkish Federation by Soran and colleagues has recently closed, and the results have not yet been published, but were presented at the 2016 ASCO Annual Meeting, which are discussed below. A US/Canadian trial (E2108) has closed accrual but not yet reported results (49). A similarly designed Phase III trial initiated by the Japan Oncology Group (JCOG 1017) is expected to close in late 2017 or early 2018 [46]. Two other trials have closed without reaching accrual; one in the Netherlands trial [47] closed with minimal accrual, while the Austrian Breast Cancer Group study (POSYTIVE, ABSCG 28, NCT01015625) closed after accruing 93 patients. Although all these studies aimed to answer similar questions, the design varied between studies in terms of timing of surgery and systemic therapy. Several require initiation of systemic therapy prior to randomization, while some randomize to up-front surgery prior to systemic therapies. See Table 6.1.

Table 6.1 Prospective randomized trials investigating the role of local-regional treatment in Stage IV breast cancer

Study	Accrual period	Accrual goal	Systemic treatment before randomization	Status	Final number of randomized patients
India	2005–12	350	Yes	Published	350
Turkey	2008–12	271	No	Presented	274
USA, Canada	2011–15	368	Yes	Closed	Projected to be 268
Japan	2011–16	500	Yes	Open	Projected to be 400
Austria	2010–19	254	No	Presented	93

6.6 Completed Trials

6.6.1 India (NCT00193778)

Badwe and colleagues in India were the first of the above groups to publish their final results. This single-institution randomized trial (RCT) at the Tata Memorial Cancer Institute in Mumbai opened for enrollment in 2005 [45]. To be eligible for randomization, patients first had to show response to systemic therapy, which was primarily six cycles of anthracycline-based chemotherapy with the addition of taxanes in 5% of patients. Of an initial 716 patients, 440 showed response to chemotherapy. Of note, only 25 of these initial 716 had surgically resectable disease before treatment. An additional 90 patients were excluded for various reasons for a final count of 350 patients eligible for randomization. They were randomized to either continue with systemic therapy alone or undergo primary site local therapy (PSLT), which consisted of surgery with or without radiation. The decision algorithm for radiotherapy was similar to that for non-metastatic patients for both breast conservation and mastectomy patients. Overall survival (OS) was the primary outcome of this trial, while secondary outcomes included locoregional progression-free survival (PFS), distant progression-free survival, and health-related quality of life.

Of the 350 patients eligible for randomization following induction systemic therapy, 177 were assigned to continue systemic therapy and 173 received PSLT before continuation of systemic therapy. Disease and demographic characteristics were well-balanced between the two groups. There were 235 deaths at the median follow-up duration of 23 months, almost equally divided between groups, with no difference in overall survival, as shown in Fig. 6.2 (HR 1.04, 95% CI 0.80–1.34). This was also true of planned subset analyses (menopausal status, bone-only disease, number of metastatic sites, hormone receptor, and HER2 status of the tumors). The secondary outcomes differed between the groups with a better locoregional PFS in the surgical group, shown in Fig. 6.3 (HR 0.16, $p = 0.001$) but better distant PFS in the systemic therapy-only group (HR 1.42, $p = 0.012$).

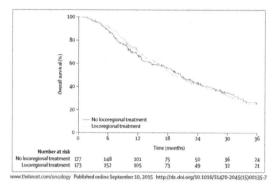

Fig. 6.2 Kaplan–Meier plot of overall survival. http://www.thelancet.com/oncology. Published online September 10, 2015 http://dx.doi.org/10.1016/S1470-2045(15)00135-7

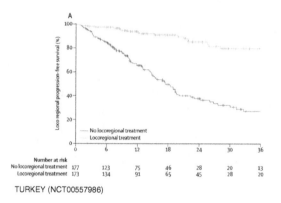

Fig. 6.3 Locoregional progression in women who did or did not recieve primary site locoregional therapy. http://www.thelancet.com/oncology. Published online September 10, 2015 http://dx.doi.org/10.1016/S1470-2045(15)00135-7

It is important to note that while recent trials have shown a median overall survival of around 40–49 months in countries where resources allow access to standard-of-care therapy [48, 49], the median survival in the India trial patients was only 19 months [45]. Additionally, among patients in the Tata Memorial group, only about 25% of the patients had three or fewer metastatic lesions, and less than a third had bone-only disease—further illuminating the advanced nature of disease in this group. Additionally, of the 90 women with HER2-positive tumors, only eight received trastuzumab as part of their systemic therapy.

6.6.2 Turkey (NCT00557986)

Unlike the Tata Memorial trial above, and the US/Canadian trial described below, the Turkish Federation trial (Protocol MF07-01) randomized de novo Stage IV patients to primary site local therapy versus systemic therapy alone [50]. While results of this trial have yet to be published, the results were presented at the 2016 American Society of Clinical Oncology (ASCO) Annual Meeting [51]. Of an initial 312 recruited patients, 274 were ultimately evaluable and included in the study, meeting their sample size calculation to achieve 90% power. Women in this study had Stage IV breast cancer at presentation and a surgically resectable primary breast tumor. The patients randomized to the PSLT group ($n = 138$) received surgery with or without radiation up front then subsequently began their systemic therapy. Patients underwent either mastectomy or breast conservation based on tumor extent and patient and physician preferences, and axillary surgery was included as for any non-metastatic patients. Axillary dissection was performed for any patients with positive sentinel nodes or needle biopsy-proven nodal disease. Free margins were required in all resections. In the end, about 75% had mastectomy and 92% had an axillary node dissection. All breast conservation patients received whole breast radiation, while postmastectomy radiation was determined based on extent of disease and institutional practice. The group randomized to systemic therapy (ST) ($n = 136$) received local therapy subsequently, if needed for palliation. Chemotherapy for both groups was primarily anthracycline-based and was similar between groups. All patients with hormone receptor-positive breast cancer received endocrine therapy, and all HER2/neu-positive patients received trastuzumab. About 30% of tumors were HER2+ in each group; however, there were more estrogen receptor-positive (ER+) tumors in the PSLT group (86%) than the ST group (73%). Surgery or radiation to distant metastatic sites was determined by physician and patient with a slightly higher rate (35%) in the ST group over the PSLT group (25%).

The primary outcome objective was overall survival (OS), and the secondary objectives were morbidity, locoregional progression/relapse, and quality of life. The primary end point was three-year survival, and this showed no significant difference in OS between the groups: HR 0.76 (95% CI 0.49–1.16), $p = 0.2$. Data with longer follow-up were presented at ASCO 2016 [51], showing a five-year OS in the surgery group of 41.6%, which was significantly higher than the 24.4% seen in the ST group ($p = 0.005$) with a hazard ratio of 0.66, 95% CI 0.49–0.88, $p = 0.005$. This translated into a nine-month longer median survival for the surgery group of 46 months compared to 37 months in the ST group.

In unplanned subset analyses, a statistically significant survival benefit from PSLT was observed in women aged less than 55 years, those with hormone receptor-positive tumors, and/or HER2-negative tumors, and those with solitary bony lesions (these were not biopsy-proven to be metastatic). Among those randomized to initial systemic therapy, those with multiple pulmonary/liver metastases appeared to fare somewhat better. Notably, only three-year survival data could be calculated for the group with multiple pulmonary/liver metastases because most of these patients died by the five-year mark. Locoregional progression/relapse was 1% ($n = 2$) in the surgery group and 11% ($n = 15$) in the ST group ($p = 0.001$). Quality of life analyses are planned.

6.6.3 Austria (NCT01015625)

The Austrian Breast and Colorectal Cancer Study Group initiated a trial (POSYTIVE) with a plan for initial randomization to locoregional therapy versus systemic therapy (45). They later amended the protocol to allow randomization of patients who had already begun systemic therapy. Those in the locoregional therapy group underwent resection of the primary and axillary surgery ± radiation and subsequently began or continued systemic therapy. Those in the systemic therapy group could undergo palliative surgical intervention later if needed. Randomization was stratified for key factors. The primary end point was overall survival, and secondary end points include time to local and distant progression. The trial experienced slow accrual and closed with 93 patients. Results were reported at the 2017 ASCO Annual Meeting, with 45 patients per arm [52]. The study arms were balanced for important variables (age, menopausal status, tumor size and intrinsic subtype, bone only versus multiple visceral ± bone, and type of systemic therapy). There was no difference in overall survival (HR 0.69, 95% CI 0.36–1.33) for the entire study population, or in specific subset analyses. Patient-reported outcomes were also reported at the same meeting, and although the surgical group reported more symptoms in the early postoperative phase, these equalized over time. A major determinant of survival was the baseline physical functioning score, which in turn was higher in women younger than 60 years of age than in those over 60.

6.7 Ongoing Trials

6.7.1 US/Canada (NCT01242800)

The US and Canadian randomized trial (E2108) was first proposed in 2002 and opened by the Eastern Cooperative Oncology Group (NCT01242800) in 2011 [53]. The initial accrual goal was 880 patients, but was lowered to 368 due to slow recruitment during the first two years. It was closed in July 2015 with 383 patients. The design required initial systemic therapy for all newly diagnosed Stage IV patients, with randomization of those with stable or responsive disease after 4–8 months of therapy. The initial therapies included endocrine, chemotherapy, or anti-HER2 agents based on tumor markers and patient factors such as menopausal status and metastatic sites, per NNCN or similar guidelines [54]. The PSLT arm received surgery and radiation therapy as would have been indicated for the same local disease in a non-metastatic setting. With a primary outcome of overall survival at three years, the study was redesigned in 2013 with power to detect a 19%

difference between groups, favoring the PSLT arm. The secondary outcomes include local progression-free survival and quality of life. Since this study will provide an excellent context for the conduct of biomarker studies exploring specific scientific hypotheses, tissue and blood samples are being banked for future-related studies.

6.7.2 Japan

As in the US/Canadian and Indian trials, the Japanese trial randomized only those women who showed at least stable disease following initial systemic therapy [46]. Initiated by the Japanese Cooperative Oncology Group (JCOG 1017), this trial began accrual in June 2011 and is expected to close in 2017. It too uses a design mandating induction systemic therapy and randomization of those who do not progress on therapy. PSLT includes resection of the primary tumor only without axillary surgery, with radiotherapy utilized only for specific indications. Overall survival is the primary end point of this trial with secondary end points including progression of distant disease, rate of uncontrolled local disease, and complications from chemotherapy or surgery. According to the trial plan published in 2012, the accrual goal is 410 randomized patients.

6.8 Prospective Registry Study

A prospective registry study has been completed in the USA, analyzing the role and utilization of surgery in patients with de novo Stage IV breast cancer, conducted by the Translational Breast Cancer Research Group (TBCRC013) [49]. The goal of this trial was to chronicle progression of local and metastatic disease in Stage IV patients, the impact of PSLT on disease progression and survival, the rate of palliative surgical resection of intact primary, and quality of life. To be eligible, patients must have been diagnosed with metastatic disease either prior to or within 3 months of primary surgery. Hundred and twenty-seven such patients from 14 institutions were accrued from 2009 to 2012. Cohort A included those with synchronous diagnosis of primary and metastatic disease, so that the primary tumor was intact at registry ($n = 112$), while cohort B comprised of those in whom metastases were found within 3 months following primary site surgery ($n = 15$).

Patients in cohort A underwent first-line systemic therapy and were assessed for response. Those with responsive or stable disease at distant sites were given the chance to discuss the option of elective surgery of their primary. Patients in cohort B had undergone resection of their primary tumor prior to diagnosis of metastatic disease, and received systemic therapy under the direction of their physician and per institutional standards.

In this observational study, 85% of cohort A patients responded to induction systemic therapy. Among responders, followed for a median of 54 months, three-year overall survival was 78%, compared to 24% for non-responders (*p*-value = 0.001). However, in this responsive group, there was no apparent benefit from PSLT (*p* = 0.85), and the lack of benefit held true regardless of tumor subtype. Progression-free survival was also not significantly different in those who underwent surgery compared to those who did not with a median time to progression of 12 versus 13 months. In addition to the above outcomes, the prognostic value of the 21-gene recurrence score (RS) in the setting of metastatic breast cancer was investigated in a preliminary analysis [55]. A high RS was found to be an independent prognostic factor for two-year OS (HR 1.83, *p* = 0.013). Furthermore, women with a high RS who were treated with initial endocrine therapy had a lower two-year survival compared with those who received chemotherapy as the first therapeutic regimen.

6.9   Conclusions

While systemic therapy has been, and will continue to be, the foundation of treatment for Stage IV breast cancer, the potential role of primary site local therapy for improving outcomes remains a subject of debate. Retrospective studies generally support a survival advantage from PSLT but are prone to significant bias and cannot on their own validate a change in practice. The first RCT, from Badwe and colleagues [45] in India, did not demonstrate a favorable impact of PSLT on survival, but did show better local disease control. Notably, these patients had quite advanced disease with most being deemed surgically unresectable at presentation. The POSYTIVE trial results, from a resource-rich environment, also show no hint of benefit for local therapy to the primary tumor, but the small size of the study is a significant limitation [52]. The prospective registry study from the TBCRC shows a similar lack of survival advantage in women receiving PSLT [49], and also suffers from a small sample size. This experience however does show the improved survival that can be achieved with contemporary, standard-of-care management of this patient group. At the same time, it highlights the importance of response to systemic therapy and again points out that non-responsive tumors are quickly lethal, so that the insertion of PSLT in this group is unlikely to convey any benefit, while carrying a burden of increased time in the hospital, potential surgical complications, and cost.

The Turkish Federation trial (MF07-0) showed no significant improvement in survival at the pre-designated primary end point of 3 years, but did show a significant survival advantage for the PSLT group at the five-year time-point with a hazard ratio of 0.67 [51]. The late appearance of this apparent advantage is surprising, and the imbalance between arms is somewhat troubling, but publication of the results may shed light on these issues. It is possible that the postulated effect of primary tumor ablation (i.e., decreasing the source for new metastatic sites) takes time to appear. Nevertheless, the treatment strategy appears to be more similar to that seen in resource-rich environments in that all participants were required to have resectable disease at entry and all patients with HER2-positive disease were treated with trastuzumab. Results from the ongoing RTCs from North America and Japan (E2108 and JCOG1017) are needed to resolve these discrepant results.

Despite conflicting results relative to overall survival, the available data are in general agreement that local progression is less frequent in women receiving PSLT; but also that local progression requiring palliative surgery is relatively rare in this population (4.5% in the TBCRC trial and 10% in the Tata Memorial trial). Therefore, initial surgery for this reason does not appear justified.

Thus with the completion of two randomized trials that reached accrual goals and one that did not, along with a prospective observational study, the clinical equipoise surrounding the question of PSLT in Stage IV breast cancer patients remains. At the moment, it appears logical to consider local therapy for the primary tumor if all sites of distant disease are well-controlled, but the primary site continues to progress—even if not yet symptomatic. The most pronounced version of this scenario is the patient with a complete response to systemic therapy at all distant sites, because they will then be categorized as Stage IV with no evaluable disease upon surgical removal of the primary tumor. Furthermore, some patients who fall into this group may reach significant long-term survival [48]. If local resection is planned, the decision for breast conservation versus mastectomy in the setting of metastatic disease should be made in much the same way as in the non-metastatic setting. As in the non-metastatic setting, there is no survival advantage from mastectomy but it does carry a higher morbidity and breast conservation should therefore be encouraged whenever anatomically feasible. As to radiation therapy, its value in this setting currently remains indeterminate. Overall, the available evidence is not yet extensive enough to support the incorporation of primary tumor radiotherapy in the treatment of de novo metastatic breast cancer; however, it may be considered following surgery on a case-by-case basis, particularly if there appears to be a high risk of quick local recurrence due to extensive local disease or involved margins. Primary radiotherapy may also be considered in selected patients since retrospective data suggest an equivalence to surgical resection.

References

1. Hortobagyi GN (2002) Can we cure limited metastatic breast cancer? J Clin Oncol 20:620–623
2. Nieto Y, Nawaz S, Jones RB et al (2002) Prognostic model for relapse after high-dose chemotherapy with autologous stem-cell transplantation for stage IV oligometastatic breast cancer. J Clin Oncol 20:707–718
3. Siegel R, Naishadham D, Jemal A (2013) Cancer statistics, 2013. CA Cancer J Clin 63:11–30
4. Andre F, Slimane K, Bachelot T et al (2004) Breast cancer with synchronous metastases: trends in survival during a 14-year period. J Clin Oncol 22:3302–3308

5. Thomas A, Khan SA, Chrischilles EA, Schroeder MC (2016) Initial surgery and survival in stage IV breast cancer in the United States, 1988–2011. JAMA Surg 151:424–431
6. Gradishar WJ, Anderson BO, Balassanian R et al (2015) Breast cancer version 2.2015. J Natl Compr Canc Netw 13:448–475
7. Khan SA (2007) Does resection of an intact breast primary improve survival in metastatic breast cancer? Oncology (Williston Park) 21:924–931
8. Bristow RE, Tomacruz RS, Armstrong DK et al (2002) Survival effect of maximal cytoreductive surgery for advanced ovarian carcinoma during the platinum era: a meta-analysis. J Clin Oncol 20:1248–1259
9. Samarasam I, Chandran BS, Sitaram V et al (2006) Palliative gastrectomy in advanced gastric cancer: is it worthwhile? ANZ J Surg 76:60–63
10. Lim S, Muhs BE, Marcus SG et al (2007) Results following resection for stage IV gastric cancer; are better outcomes observed in selected patient subgroups? J Surg Oncol 95:118–122
11. Ruo L, Gougoutas C, Paty PB et al (2003) Elective bowel resection for incurable stage IV colorectal cancer: prognostic variables for asymptomatic patients. J Am Coll Surg 196:722–728
12. Flanigan RC, Salmon SE, Blumenstein BA et al (2001) Nephrectomy followed by interferon alfa-2b compared with interferon alfa-2b alone for metastatic renal-cell cancer. N Engl J Med 345:1655–1659
13. Mickisch GH, Garin A, van PH et al (2001) Radical nephrectomy plus interferon-alfa-based immunotherapy compared with interferon alfa alone in metastatic renal-cell carcinoma: a randomised trial. Lancet 358:966–970
14. Chang SJ, Hodeib M, Chang J, Bristow RE (2013) Survival impact of complete cytoreduction to no gross residual disease for advanced-stage ovarian cancer: a meta-analysis. Gynecol Oncol 130:493–498
15. Comen EA (2012) Tracking the seed and tending the soil: evolving concepts in metastatic breast cancer. Discov Med 14:97–104
16. Norton L, Massague J (2006) Is cancer a disease of self-seeding? Nat Med 12:875–878
17. Karnoub AE, Dash AB, Vo AP et al (2007) Mesenchymal stem cells within tumour stroma promote breast cancer metastasis. Nature 449:557–563
18. Danna EA, Sinha P, Gilbert M et al (2004) Surgical removal of primary tumor reverses tumor-induced immunosuppression despite the presence of metastatic disease. Cancer Res 64:2205–2211
19. Gunduz N, Fisher B, Saffer EA (1979) Effect of surgical removal on the growth and kinetics of residual tumor. Cancer Res 39:3861–3865
20. Fisher B, Gunduz N, Coyle J et al (1989) Presence of a growth-stimulating factor in serum following primary tumor removal in mice. Cancer Res 49:1996–2001
21. Perletti G, Concari P, Giardini R et al (2000) Antitumor activity of endostatin against carcinogen-induced rat primary mammary tumors. Cancer Res 60:1793–1796
22. Khan SA, Stewart AK, Morrow M (2002) Does aggressive local therapy improve survival in metastatic breast cancer? Surgery 132:620–626
23. Rapiti E, Verkooijen HM, Vlastos G et al (2006) Complete excision of primary breast tumor improves survival of patients with metastatic breast cancer at diagnosis. J Clin Oncol 24:2743–2749
24. Gnerlich JJ, D.B., A.D. D, Beers C et al (2007) Surgical removal of the primary tumor increases overall survival in patients with metastatic breast cancer: analysis of the 1988–2003 SEER data. Ann Surg Oncol 14(8):2187–2194
25. Ruiterkamp J, Ernst MF, LV vdP-F et al (2009) Surgical resection of the primary tumour is associated with improved survival in patients with distant metastatic breast cancer at diagnosis. Eur J Surg Oncol 35(11):1146–1151. doi:10.1016/j.ejso.2009.03.012
26. Dominici L, Najita J, Hughes M et al (2011) Surgery of the primary tumor does not improve survival in stage IV breast cancer. Breast Cancer Res Treat 129:459–465

27. Babiera GV, Rao R, Feng L et al (2006) Effect of primary tumor extirpation in breast cancer patients who present with stage IV disease and an intact primary tumor. Ann Surg Oncol 13:776–782

28. Rao R, Feng L, Kuerer HM et al (2008) Timing of surgical intervention for the intact primary in stage IV breast cancer patients. Ann Surg Oncol 15:1696–1702

29. Neuman HB, Morrogh M, Gonen M et al (2010) Stage IV breast cancer in the era of targeted therapy: does surgery of the primary tumor matter? Cancer 116:1226–1233

30. Barkley CR, Bafford AC, Burstein HJ et al (2007) Breast surgery for women presenting with stage IV breast cancer. In: Breast cancer research and treatment SABCS 2007

31. Blanchard DK, Shetty PB, Hilsenbeck SG, Elledge RM (2008) Association of surgery with improved survival in stage IV breast cancer patients. Ann Surg 247:732–738

32. Hazard HW, Gorla SR, Kim J et al (2007) Surgical resection of the primary tumor in stage IV breast cancer and survival. Surg Oncol 14:1–128

33. Fields RC, Jeffe DB, Trinkaus K et al (2007) Surgical resection of the primary tumor is associated with increased long-term survival in patients with stage IV breast cancer after controlling for site of metastasis. Ann Surg Oncol 14(12):3345–3351

34. Leung AM, Vu HN, Nguyen KA et al (2010) Effects of surgical excision on survival of patients with stage IV breast cancer. J Surg Res 161:83–88

35. Shien T, Kinoshita T, Shimizu C et al (2009) Primary tumor resection improves the survival of younger patients with metastatic breast cancer. Oncol Rep 21:827–832

36. Pathy NB, Verkooijen HM, Taib NA et al (2011) Impact of breast surgery on survival in women presenting with metastatic breast cancer. Br J Surg 98:1566–1572

37. Le Scodan R, Stevens D, Brain E et al (2009) Breast cancer with synchronous metastases: survival impact of exclusive locoregional radiotherapy. J Clin Oncol 27:1375–1381

38. Nguyen DH, Truong PT, Alexander C et al (2012) Can locoregional treatment of the primary tumor improve outcomes for women with stage IV breast cancer at diagnosis? Int J Radiat Oncol Biol Phys 84:39–45

39. Perez-Fidalgo JA, Pimentel P, Caballero A et al (2011) Removal of primary tumor improves survival in metastatic breast cancer. Does timing of surgery influence outcomes? Breast 20:548–554

40. Cady B, Nathan NR, Michaelson JS et al (2008) Matched pair analyses of stage IV breast cancer with or without resection of primary breast site. Ann Surg Oncol 15:3384–3395

41. Ruiterkamp J, Voogd AC, Bosscha K et al (2011) Presence of symptoms and timing of surgery do not affect the prognosis of patients with primary metastatic breast cancer. Eur J Surg Oncol 37:883–889

42. Hazard HW, Gorla SR, Scholtens D et al. (2008) Surgical resection of the primary tumor, chest wall control, and survival in women with metastatic breast cancer. Cancer 15:113 (8):2011–2019. doi:10.1002/cncr.23870

43. Hartmann S, Reimer T, Gerber B, Stachs A (2014) Primary metastatic breast cancer: the impact of locoregional therapy. Breast Care (Basel) 9:23–28

44. Ruiterkamp J, Voogd AC, Bosscha K et al (2011) Presence of symptoms and timing of surgery do not affect the prognosis of patients with primary metastatic breast cancer. Eur J Surg Oncol 37:883–889

45. Badwe R, Hawaldar R, Nair N et al (2015) Locoregional treatment versus no treatment of the primary tumour in metastatic breast cancer: an open-label randomised controlled trial. Lancet Oncol 16:1380–1388

46. Shien T, Nakamura K, Shibata T et al (2012) A randomized controlled trial comparing primary tumour resection plus systemic therapy with systemic therapy alone in metastatic breast cancer (PRIM-BC): Japan Clinical Oncology Group Study JCOG1017. Jpn J Clin Oncol 42:970–973

47. Ruiterkamp J, Voogd AC, Tjan-Heijnen VC et al (2012) SUBMIT: systemic therapy with or without up front surgery of the primary tumor in breast cancer patients with distant metastases at initial presentation. BMC Surg 12:5

48. Cardoso F, Costa A, Norton L et al (2014) ESO-ESMO 2nd international consensus guidelines for advanced breast cancer (ABC2). Breast 23:489–502

49. King TA LJ, Gonen M et al (2016) A prospective analysis of surgery and survival in stage IV breast cancer. In J Clin Oncol; ASCO annual conference 2016. Annual Meeting June 4, 2016: Abstract 1006

50. Soran A, Ozbas S, Kelsey SF, Gulluoglu BM (2009) Randomized trial comparing locoregional resection of primary tumor with no surgery in stage IV breast cancer at the presentation (Protocol MF07-01): a study of Turkish Federation of the National Societies for Breast Diseases. Breast J 15:399–403

51. Soran A OV, Ozbas S et al (2016) A randomized controlled trial evaluating resection of the primary breast tumor in women presenting with de novo stage IV breast cancer. J Clin Oncol; 34 ASCO 2016. Annual Meeting June 4, 2016: Abstract 176

52. Fitzal FGM, Steger G, Singer CF, Marth C, Hubalek M et al (2017) Primary operation in synchronous metastasized breast cancer patients: first oncologic outcomes of the prospective randomized phase III ABCSG28 POSYTIVE trial. In: ASCO Chicago 2017. Annual Meeting June 3, 2017: Abstract 1074

53. Perez CB, Khan SA (2011) Local therapy for the primary breast tumor in women with metastatic disease. Clin Adv Hematol Oncol 9:112–119

54. Theriault RL, Carlson RW, Allred C et al (2013) Breast cancer, version 3.2013: featured updates to the NCCN guidelines. J Natl Compr Canc Netw 11:753–760; quiz 761

55. King TA, Lyman JP, Gonen M et al (2016) Prognostic impact of 21-gene recurrence score in patients with stage IV breast cancer: TBCRC 013. J Clin Oncol 34:2359–2365

Advancements and Personalization of Breast Cancer Treatment Strategies in Radiation Therapy

Meena S. Moran

7

Contents

Abstract

Significant technologic advances in radiation treatment delivery now allow for more personalized delivery considerations which incorporate individual patient characteristics (such as tumor location and patient anatomy) and more precise delivery in the breast conservation or post-mastectomy setting. The combined

M. S. Moran (✉)
Therapeutic Radiology, Yale Radiation Therapy Program,
Yale University School of Medicine, New Haven, USA
e-mail: meena.moran@yale.edu

© Springer International Publishing AG 2018
W. J. Gradishar (ed.), *Optimizing Breast Cancer Management*, Cancer Treatment
and Research 173, https://doi.org/10.1007/978-3-319-70197-4_7

advancements with other treatment modalities (i.e., systemic therapy, surgical management) have had direct effects on local-regional management and outcomes such that currently, local-regional relapses after definitive treatment for localized disease are now rarely experienced. Recent advances in the radiation therapy field have come from careful patient selection for a variety of three-dimensional treatment delivery techniques and alternatives to conventional tangential radiation. These advances have been demonstrated to diminished acute/long-term toxicity, minimized dose to surrounding normal tissue structures such as the heart and lung, and ultimately result in an improvement in the therapeutic ratio for radiation treatment. This chapter discusses recent radiation innovations and appropriate patient selection for their application, for a more personalized approach to radiation therapy for breast cancer patients.

Keywords

Breast cancer · Radiation therapy · Techniques · Deep inspiration breath hold · Breast conservation therapy · Regional nodal radiation

7.1 Introduction

Breast conservation therapy (BCT) remains the standard alternative to mastectomy for early-stage disease established by multiple trials initiated more than two decades ago [1–5]. Since the era in which these trials were conducted, multiple advances in screening, surgical techniques, pathologic handling, systemic treatment options, and classification of tumors into prognostic biologic sub-types have all contributed to the ultimate resulted in detection of breast cancers at earlier, more favorable stages of disease [6], and better overall outcomes [1, 2, 4, 6]. The mainstream use of biologic sub-typing and gene assays to stratify individual recurrence risk have significantly helped to identify which patients may benefit from more versus less systemic treatment [7, 8]. The development and widespread use of systemic agents including a variety of new endocrine receptor modulators, additional targeted agents against HER2-positive disease, and routine use of anthracyclines and taxanes have, beyond providing the intended direct improvements in distant disease-free and overall survival outcomes, resulted in the inadvertent effects of further reducing local-regional relapse (LRR) beyond the effects of seen with radiation therapy [9]. Within the field of radiation therapy, significant technologic advances in treatment delivery now allow for more personalized delivery considerations which incorporate individual patient characteristics (such as tumor location and patient anatomy) and more precise delivery of radiation in the breast conservation or post-mastectomy setting. Unlike the conventional tangential beams that were utilized in the earlier BCT and post-mastectomy radiation therapy (PMRT) trials, significant advancements in planning and delivery now routinely incorporate three-dimensional techniques that result in a more uniform delivery of the dose across the targeted volume, which has resulted in significantly decreasing both acute and long-term skin toxicities and decreased the exposure and toxicity to surrounding critical normal tissue such as heart, lung, and contralateral breast. These simultaneous improvements in radiation techniques, together with the above-mentioned advances, have produced excellent local-regional control with contemporary treatment such that local-regional relapses after definitive treatment for localized disease are rare. Hence, the combined multi-modality effects on local-regional control and the diminished acute/long-term toxicity from advances in radiation techniques have resulted in an improvement in the therapeutic ratio for radiation treatment. As such, the role of adjuvant radiation in the management of breast cancer is rapidly evolving. Better stratification of individual patients' risk versus benefit ratio for local-regional recurrence and distant disease will allow for selection of low-risk subsets who may forgo traditional radiation for lesser or no radiation treatments, and those at higher risk who may warrant a more aggressive approach with inclusion of regional nodal radiation.

In this chapter, recent advancements in radiation therapy delivery techniques and their applications for selected patients are reviewed. Treatment modalities such as partial breast irradiation, hypo-fractionated whole breast radiation, and specific techniques for decreasing toxicity are discussed. Considerations for post-mastectomy radiation and regional nodal radiation are evaluated. Lastly, review of recent data to support omission of radiation after breast-conserving surgery in low-risk subsets is discussed.

7.2 Hypo-fractionated Whole Breast Radiation

The most important advancement in the twentieth century in the field of breast radiation oncology has been the routine adoption of BCT for preservation of the breast in early-stage breast cancer. The early prospective, randomized trials of BCT all utilized standard, two-dimensional tangential WBRT after local excision of the primary tumor, and consistently demonstrated the benefits of WBRT in decreasing ipsilateral breast tumor recurrence (IBTR) when added to breast-conserving surgery alone [1–5]. More recently, the Early Breast Cancer Trialists' Collaborative Group meta-analysis of the randomized studies, with over 7300 patients, has changed the paradigm that radiation only effects local-regional relapse, by demonstrating the small but statistically significant benefit that WBRT contributes to overall survival [10]. The vast majority of patients treated in the original BCT trials received WBRT to doses of 45–50 Gy in 25–28 fractions delivered over a period of 5–6 weeks, with a more recent practice of delivering a boost to the lumpectomy bed further extending the delivery time to 6–7 weeks. Thus, a major disadvantage with WBRT is the prolonged treatment course and its potential for convenience for patients. Ultimately, only 2/3 of patients receive postoperative radiotherapy after breast-conserving surgery despite its well-established benefits, and the utilization of BCT is not been uniform with marked variation in the use of BCT by geographic region [11, 12]. There are also data suggesting that longer distance to radiation therapy centers acts as a deterrent for utilization of standard radiation treatment courses [13, 14].

The rationale for using conventional fractionation (small daily fractions to a high total dose) is based on theoretic radiobiological modeling that has historically suggested that the vast majority of tumors have relatively low sensitivity to changes in daily fraction size, whereas normal tissues generally have a higher relative sensitivity to changes in radiation fraction size [15]. Conventional fractionation has taken advantage of the difference in sensitivity of normal and tumor cells to fraction size, so that at lower radiation fractions, damage to normal tissue is less than the damage to tumor cells. More contemporary radiobiological evidence has shown that, in fact, normal breast tissue and breast tumors have very similar sensitivity to dose fraction size. And if so, then there may no longer be an added therapeutic advantage in delivering smaller daily fraction sizes for reducing toxicity [16].

With the discovery that the standard assumptions for fractionation derived originally from several epithelial tumors do not pertain to breast tumors, several randomized trials have been conducted to utilize larger daily fraction sizes in breast cancer to shorten the radiation treatment course. We now have mature data consistently establishing the equivalence of hypo-fractionated and conventionally fractionated WBRT [17–21]. Thus, the use of moderately hypo-fractionated radiotherapy using schedules such as 40 Gy delivered in 15 fractions over 3 weeks is now considered as efficacious and safe as conventionally fractionated WBRT for many patients after breast-conserving surgery (with or without incorporation of the boost, Fig. 7.1), though for selected subgroups, such as those of younger age, patients receiving neoadjuvant or adjuvant chemotherapy, or those who require regional nodal radiotherapy, additional data are needed. Of note, only a small minority of patients on these hypo-fractionation trials received regional nodal irradiation, were treated in the post-mastectomy setting, or received a radiation therapy boost to the tumor bed.

Based on a review of these data, American Society of Radiation Oncology (ASTRO) published a guideline recommending hypo-fractionated whole breast radiation for patients who are 50 years or older, considered for breast tangential radiation with tumors that are pT1-2 pN0 (therefore no regional nodal radiation), who have not received chemotherapy, for whom a radiation plan can be generated with a radiation dose homogeneity within ±7% in the central axis plane. Within this guideline, it is stated that for all other patients not meeting these criteria, the data are limited since these subgroups were relatively underrepresented on these trials [22]. One of the three breast 'Choosing Wisely' campaigns for ASTRO has been 'Do not initiate WBRT as a part of BCT in women age ≥ 50 with early-stage invasive breast cancer without considering shorter treatment schedules.' Based on phase III trials that have now demonstrated equivalent tumor control and cosmetic outcomes in specific patient populations using shorter fractionation schedules of approximately 3–4 weeks. Thus, patients and their physicians should discuss the option of hypo-fractionation WBRT to determine the most appropriate course of therapy [23].

Additionally, the results of ongoing additional trials may allow for even shorter radiation schemas. There are currently several trials assessing the efficacy and safety of faster-accelerated WBRT schedules. For example, in the UK, the FAST FORWARD trial is assessing their national standard of 3-week WBRT against a 1-week course of WBRT. While long-term outcomes for the 4000 patients

Weeks: Standard Fractionation of Treatment:

Whole Breast Radiation Plus Boost to Tumor Bed

Whole Breast Radiation (No boost)

Weeks: Hypofractionated Fractionation

Whole Breast Radiation Plus Boost to Tumor Bed

Whole Breast Radiation (No boost)

Weeks: Accelerated Partial Breast Irradiation

Multi-luminal Brachytherapy, intracavity brachytherapy, 3D CRT APBI

Days: Intra-operative Accelerated Partial Breast Irradiation

Electron or Kilovotage beams

Observation: Omission of RT

Fig. 7.1 Schematic representation demonstrating standard fractionation with and without boost, hypo-fractionation with and without boost, and accelerated partial breast irradiation. Alternatively, selected patients may be candidates for omission of adjuvant radiation therapy

enrolled on this trial are awaited, a recent sub-study analysis from this cohort reported that the acute skin toxicity conducted in patients entered into this trial was mild and raised no concerns [14]. Protocols exploring hypo-fractionation in the post-mastectomy radiation therapy and post-systemic therapy settings are also underway, and ultimately, should result in an expansion of the indications for the use of hypo-fractionated radiation for breast cancer.

7.3 Accelerated Partial Breast Irradiation (APBI)

APBI typically involves treatment of a three-dimensional volume that includes a margin of several centimeters around the lumpectomy cavity, which is the region at highest risk for IBTR. The advantage of APBI, in addition to typically rapid (1 week or less, Fig. 7.1) treatment delivery, is the potential for significant sparing of normal, unaffected breast tissue from high-dose radiation. The rationale for APBI is supported by both clinical and pathologic data suggesting that the benefit of radiotherapy results from the eradication of microscopic disease immediately adjacent to the lumpectomy cavity [24]. Data from several prospective and retrospective trials indicate that most IBTRs occur within or immediately adjacent to the lumpectomy bed [25–27], with only 4% or less of IBTR occurring in regions remote from the original tumor bed [28, 29]. Therefore, the benefit of postoperative radiotherapy in diminishing local relapse may still be attainable while treating a smaller volume of tissue and sparing high dose radiation to the entire breast. By treating larger daily fractions to a partial breast volume, the patient can theoretically achieve the local control of radiation with the added benefits of increased convenience due to the shorter delivery period, and potentially have less side effects due to sparing to unaffected normal breast tissue.

There are several general categories of techniques for delivering APBI, which include interstitial brachytherapy, single-lumen or multiple-lumen balloon-based high-dose-rate brachytherapy, 3D conformal radiation therapy (3D-CRT), and intraoperative radiotherapy (IORT). The existing published data on APBI come from retrospective, single-institution, or single-arm prospective series and the published randomized prospective studies comparing APBI with WBRT are limited. Notably, the longest follow-up comes from institutions with significant expertise in intraluminal brachytherapy techniques, which are known to be user-dependent and require meticulous and skilled placement of catheters in the lumpectomy bed. The longest follow-up for APBI comes from multi-catheter brachytherapy experience, with these long-term data suggesting that in highly selected, low-risk patients, the use of brachytherapy techniques may be a safe and efficacious alternative to WBRT (Fig. 7.2). Given the high user-dependence and significant learning curve for interstitial brachytherapy catheter placement, the availability of this delivery modality for APBI has been limited to radiation centers with this specific expertise [30–32].

Intraluminal brachytherapy (or balloon brachytherapy) was rapidly incorporated into the clinics with widespread marketing that boasted a simpler, less operator-dependent delivery of APBI, with the added advantages of reproducible

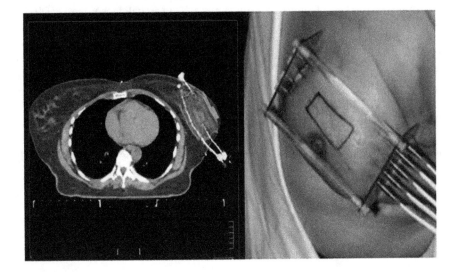

Fig. 7.2 Left image shows CT scan with catheters in place after lumpectomy, with dose distribution of the APBI volume. Right image shows one of several techniques of catheters placed through lumpectomy cavity

dosimetry and improved comfort for patients than with the multi-catheter brachytherapy technique [15]. This technique makes use of a silicone balloon connected to a catheter that is placed into the lumpectomy cavity intraoperatively after definitive surgery. The balloon is inflated with saline and contrast, and a computed tomography (CT) scan is performed to document adequate device positioning to enable treatment planning. Postoperatively, the patient is brought to the radiation department where an HDR Ir-192 source is remotely after-loaded into the catheter, delivering two fractions daily over five days. The widespread use of intraluminal brachytherapy preceded the data to support its use. Ultimately, the American Society of Breast Surgeons (ASBS) developed a MammoSite™ (Hologic, Bedford, MA) registry and users from nearly 100 institutions across the USA entered patient information (before, during, or after treatment) for future analysis of delivery, local relapse, and cosmesis parameters. The MammoSite™ registry has now provided a large body of data with adequate follow-up to suggest its safety and efficacy in selected patient subgroups [33–35]. To address the inherent limitations in dose shaping using a single lumen, particularly with lesions that are close to the skin or chest wall, where an increased risk of fat necrosis and severe skin toxicity is reported, devices have subsequently been developed with multiple-lumen catheters, which allow for improved dosimetry by providing more source placement options to improve dose conformation [15].

One of the most popular and appealing forms of APBI has been three-dimensional conformal radiotherapy (3D-CRT) because of its inherent requirement for utilization of EBRT technology which is well understood and available to most radiation oncologist, and lack of need for specific dedicated equipment for APBI. Compared with standard tangential techniques, 3D-CRT APBI with linear accelerator-generated X-ray beams often results in higher normal tissue doses than other APBI techniques, (Fig. 7.3) which raises some concerns for increase in long-term toxicity. For example, one concern of 3D-CRT is the potential for increased long-term toxicity from the larger volume of breast tissue around the tumor bed (relative to brachytherapy-based APBI methods) that is needed with 3D-CRT/IMRT APBI to account for respiration, patient motion, and set-up errors. In addition, the use of multiple-beam configurations inevitably exposes a much larger volume of normal tissue (i.e., lungs, ribs, and contralateral breast) to low-dose radiation, which can potentially result in increased in long-term toxicity (Fig. 7.3). Although some studies, such as the RTOG (Radiation Therapy Oncology Group) 0319, a prospective single-arm phase II trial, and interim analysis of NSABP B39/RTOG 0413, both report minimal toxicity using 3D CRT APBI [36, 37], other published data suggest that 3D CRT APBI may be associated with unacceptable long-term cosmesis or result in significantly worse fibrosis than that experienced with whole breast radiation techniques [38–40].

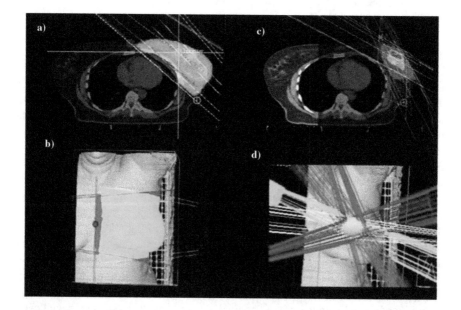

Fig. 7.3 Dose distribution and beam arrangements of whole breast radiation (WBRT) versus accelerated partial breast irradiation (APBI) using linear accelerator-generated 3D/IMRT techniques. Green depicts the high-dose region. **a** The dose distribution of a WBRT tangential plan using a field-in-field technique (FIF-3D). **b** Digital reconstruction of the treatment planning scan showing the projection of the beams over the skin for WBRT. **c** The dose distribution depicting a 3D/IMRT APBI plan using multiple beams to target the lumpectomy cavity with a 2 cm margin. **d** Digital reconstruction of the treatment planning scan showing the projection of the beams over the skin for APBI

Lastly, intraoperative APBI methods are also commercially available which allow a mobile treatment device to deliver a single, one-time fraction of approximately 20 Gy intraoperatively to the tumor bed using electrons or low-energy X-rays. The advantages of intraoperative targeting include the reduction of the possibility of a geographic miss, the convenience of one treatment, and significant reductions in cost. A major disadvantage is the lack of final pathology (i.e., margin status) at the time of radiation delivery, which is critical in guiding decisions regarding patient selection decisions for APBI. For a variety of reasons, the trials exploring intraoperative APBI have been met with significant controversy [41–44].

One of the fastest accruing trials for breast cancer in the field of radiation therapy has been the Radiation Therapy Oncology Group (RTOG) 0413/National Surgical Adjuvant Breast and Bowel Project (NSABP) B-39 phase III trial, which randomized patients to APBI versus WBRT, with the APBI technique (i.e., interstitial, lumen-based, or three-dimensional external beam-based) chosen at the discretion of the treating physician. Long-term results are not expected for several more years. Yet, despite lack of mature data from randomized trials, the use of APBI has been rapidly increasing, both on and off protocol, in large academic centers as well as community-based hospitals and private practice settings, due to the enthusiasm for the relative shorter fractionation schemas, which range from intraoperative APBI delivered in 1 day (on the day of lumpectomy), to 3D/IMRT external beam and brachytherapy methods, which typically allow the entire course to be delivered in less than 1 week. This enthusiasm has been compounded by widespread marketing for APBI proceeding level 1 data to support its use.

In order to guide patient selection and promote best practices for APBI while awaiting results for long-term data from randomized trials, the American Society for Therapeutic Radiology and Oncology (ASTRO) initially published an APBI guideline in 2009, separating patients into three categories of suitable, cautionary, and unsuitable for APBI [45]. The suitable group includes patients in whom data from phase II studies exist supporting the use of APBI and includes those low-risk patients for whom WBRT would be unlikely to confer a survival benefit. The cautionary and unsuitable groups represent patient subgroups for whom these are minimal data to support APBI and in whom WBRT has been demonstrated to provide a survival benefit. With preliminary results of randomized trials and longer follow-up from previously reported series, ASTRO has recently updated the APBI guideline [46]. Significant changes to the updated consensus statement include recommendations to lower the minimum age of women considered 'suitable' for APBI from the previously recommended age of 60 years to 50 years, in addition to including subsets of patients with ductal carcinoma in situ with low/intermediate grade, $\leq$2.5 cm, negative surgical margins. Of note, patients 40 years or older who meet all other suitability requirements, including patients with low-risk DCIS, are considered 'cautionary' candidates for APBI. With regard to intraoperative APBI methods, the guideline specifies that based on data with 5.8-year median follow-up [42], the low-energy X-ray IORT should be used only in the context of a prospective registry or clinical trial and should be restricted to women with invasive cancers who are considered otherwise deemed suitable for partial breast irradiation.

Given the critical effects of WBRT on overall survival, it is important to remember that long-term (≥ 15-year) follow-up is mandatory to fully appreciate any effects of local recurrence on survival and toxicity outcomes; hence, the median follow-up times currently reported in the existing published PIII trials remain insufficient for drawing meaningful conclusions. APBI is a heterogeneous treatment approach with diverse delivery techniques, each with its own complex sets of clinical, technical, and dosimetric considerations. It is highly likely that as data from clinical trials mature, current recommendations will continue to evolve to refine patient subgroups who can be safely treated with APBI.

7.4 Omission of Whole Breast Radiation After Breast-Conserving Surgery: Early-Stage Invasive Cancer

The standard for early-stage invasive cancer remains breast-conserving surgery to attain negative margins (defined as no ink on tumor) [47] followed by WBRT as the alternative to mastectomy. Despite data suggesting that WBRT after BCS decreases local relapse consistently across all age groups and pathologic characteristics, it is likely that there are subgroups of patients in whom the more indolent natural history of their disease may allow for omission of WBRT. It is important to note that, to date, all patient subgroups in the original BCT trials appear to benefit from adjuvant WBRT and, to date, no patient subgroups have been consistently identified in whom WBRT does not result in a statistically significant benefit in decreasing local relapse. Nevertheless, for certain low-risk subgroups with favorable, small tumors in whom the benefit in local control may not translate into a small long-term survival benefit, the routine utilization of radiation has been questioned.

Specifically for the elderly breast cancer population, who inherently have shorter life expectancies, were under-represented in the original breast conservation therapy trials (with many of the protocols excluding patients ≥ 70 years of age) and often have competing comorbidities, there has been active investigation of omitting WBRT in selected low-risk elderly subgroups. There are now several prospective randomized trials that change the paradigm of routine WBRT after BCT for elderly patients. Two of these studies, the CALGB 9343 and the PRIME II, randomized 'elderly' patients with low-risk, hormone receptor-positive disease to WBRT with hormone therapy versus close observation with hormone therapy (no WBRT). The CALGB 9343 included women ≥ 70 years with tumors ≤ 2 cm, who were *clinically* node-negative and ER-positive and received tamoxifen [48], whereas PRIME II trial included patients ≥ 65 years with tumors ≤ 3 cm in size with primarily grade I/II disease, all estrogen receptor ER-positive and pathologically node-negative [49]. Each of these studies similarly reported acceptable local relapse rates for both cohorts treated with or without whole breast radiation therapy (PRIME II 5-year rate of 4.1% no WBRT vs. 1.3% with WBRT, $p = 0.0002$;

CALGB 9343 10-year rate of 10% no WBRT vs. 2% with WBRT, $p < 0.001$) [49, 50]. Though these differences in local relapse between the arms of each study were statistically significant, the addition of whole breast radiation therapy did not result in differences in axillary recurrence, distant metastasis, or breast cancer-specific survival. In fact, the majority of deaths in both the PRIME II and CALGB trials were non-breast cancer-related events.

In addition, omission of WBRT has been explored in other subsets perceived to be at low risk for local relapse. For example, the 2×2 designed randomized BASO II trial included 1135 women aged <70 years, with the median age of 57 years (range, 33–69 years). The study reported 10-year local control of 93% with WBRT versus 93% for the tamoxifen-alone arm ($p = 0.90$). However, patients who had received WBRT + tamoxifen arm had local control of 100% which dropped significantly to 83% for patients who received no tamoxifen and no WBRT [51].

Together, these data suggest that in highly selected subsets of low-risk patients such as those older than 65 or 70 years with hormone receptor-positive disease and/or other favorable factors, breast cancer-specific survival is not affected by the omission of WBRT. Based on these data, the National Comprehensive Cancer Network (NCCN) currently recommends that omission of WBRT may be considered in patients ≥ 70 years of age with ER-positive, clinically node-negative, T1 tumors who receive adjuvant endocrine therapy (category 1 evidence) [52]. Recently, a study using the National Cancer Institute—Surveillance, Epidemiology, and End Results (SEER) database to compare use of radiation in a low-risk elderly population ≥ 70 years old from 2000 to 2004 (pre-CALGB 9343) versus 2005 to 2009 (post-CALGB) demonstrated that use of radiation therapy declined by <7% (from 68.6% pre-CALGB to 61.7% post-CALGB, $p < 0.001$). Though the use of external beam radiotherapy specifically went down from 66 to 54% ($p < 0.001$), an unexpected and fascinating finding was a simultaneous increase in implant-based radiotherapy from 1.4 to 6.2%, which diminished the overall effect of omitting radiation in these low-risk elderly patients [53].

Over time, it is likely that other low-risk subgroups will be identified in whom WBRT can be omitted safely without compromising breast cancer-specific outcomes. Ultimately, the decision to omit radiotherapy is complex and multifactorial, resulting from concerns related to length of treatment, convenience, cost, access to care, geographic variations, ethnicity-based differences, physician biases, and most importantly, patient preferences.

7.5 Omission of Whole Breast Radiation After Breast-Conserving Surgery: Ductal Carcinoma in Situ (DCIS)

Though the standard of care for localized DCIS remains breast-conserving surgery to attain negative margins (defined as ≥ 2 mm) [54] followed by WBRT, the optimal management strategies for DCIS continue to be increasingly controversial, in light of the breast cancer-specific survival for DCIS which approaches nearly 100%, irrespective of local treatment choice, in addition to the absence of level 1 data demonstrating any direct effects of treatment on overall survival. Similar to invasive cancers, an area of active research has been to attempt to identify subsets of DCIS patients in whom WBRT may be omitted. To date, subgroups of DCIS patients for whom WBRT has not been beneficial in decreasing invasive in-breast recurrences have yet to be consistently defined. One of the largest controversies is defining the primary endpoint and goal(s) of treatment, since treating physicians do not agree whether it should be *all* in-breast recurrences, irrespective of invasive or in situ, (because any recurrence is generally very meaningful for the patient), or alternatively, whether it should be the measurement of only invasive events, which theoretically have the potential to metastasize and ultimately affect survival. Based on disease estimates from the long-term follow-up of the four randomized DCIS radiation trials, the 15-year in-breast recurrence with local excision alone across the whole spectrum of DCIS ranged between 20 and 30+%, which is decreased to 10–15% with WBRT, and is well under 10% with tamoxifen at 15 years [55–58]. Of these, less than 50% are invasive recurrences. Thus, radiation oncologists often use '<1% per year' for a rule-of-thumb threshold for an acceptable upper limit of in-breast recurrences with breast radiation therapy [59], though these numbers may in fact be an over-representation of local relapse in the current era, given the improvements in pathologic handling, margin assessments, and more recent advancements in screening/earlier detection.

The only contemporary, prospective, phase III trial assessing omission of WBRT in low-risk DCIS is the RTOG 98-04, which randomized mammographically detected grade I/II DCIS measuring <2.5 cm treated with local excision and margins >3 mm to either WBRT versus observation. Tamoxifen receipt was documented as 62% of the entire cohort. Despite premature closing of the trial due to poor accrual with only one-third of its projected enrollment ($n = 636$ of 1800), the initial 7-year analysis demonstrated a significantly greater risk of in-breast recurrences for patients who did not receive WBRT (7% vs. ≤ 1%; $p < 0.001$), leading the authors to conclude that despite the perception of low-risk DCIS with widely negative margins and despite the limited number of events and underpowered sample size, WBRT nevertheless significantly reduced the number of in-breast events, and longer follow-up was needed because of the protracted clinical course of DCIS [60].

Two other prospective, single-arm studies assessed omission of WBRT for 'low-risk' DCIS. The first study, named 'The Wide local Excision Alone' (The WEA Study), defined as mammographically detected 'low-risk' DCIS lesions

<2.5 cm in size with ≥10 mm margins and predominantly grade I/II. Tamoxifen was not delivered. This trial closed early due to the extraordinarily high number of in-breast events that met the protocol's stopping rules ($n = 158$). At 5 years, the cumulative incidence of in-breast recurrence of 12% (annual recurrence rate of 2.4% per year) [61]. The more recent 10-year update reported a cumulative incidence of 15.6%, leading the authors to conclude that the risk of local relapse increases over time and remains substantial for favorable DCIS treated with wide excision margins without radiation with longer follow-up [62].

The other prospective study, ECOG 5194, was a single-arm evaluation of two separate 'low-risk' cohort. The protocol specified margins ≥3 mm in all patients and required sequential sectioning and complete embedding of each specimen, a practice which is not routine in many institutions. Each of the two cohorts was distinguished by its grade and size, with cohort 1 defined as low/intermediate grade, larger (up to 2.5 cm) size and cohort 2 defined as high grade, smaller (≤1 cm) tumors. The initial analysis at 5 years reported in-breast recurrences of 6.1% for cohort 1 and 15.3% for cohort 2, leading the authors to initially conclude that recurrences in cohort 2 were too high to consider surgery alone, but that it was reasonable to consider omitting radiation for patients with pathologic characteristics of Group 1 [63]. However, the more recent 12-year update demonstrated in-breast recurrences steadily increased over time for both cohorts, with in-breast recurrences of 14.4% and 24.6% for cohorts 1 and 2, respectively. Of these, approximately 50% was invasive (13.4% and 7.5%, respectively) as expected. At this publication, due to the steady increase in local relapse without plateau for these seemingly low-risk patients, the authors retracted the initial conclusion that omission of WBRT was reasonable for DCIS patients with pathologic characteristics of cohort 1, and revised the conclusion to state that these data were a starting point for beginning discussions in the treatment decision process [64].

Collectively, these data suggest that the natural history of DCIS is protracted, with the overall (absolute) risk for in-breast recurrence increasing over time. Unfortunately, the current methods of identifying low-risk DCIS, whether clinical-pathologic criteria or genomic testing, are not truly identifying those with indolent disease [65]. While these advances may allow for separation of the wide spectrum of DCIS into smaller subgroups in which the absolute risk of in-breast relapse is lower, a significant proportion will develop in-breast (and invasive) recurrences, and, to date, WBRT remains beneficial in significantly reducing these recurrences in all DCIS subgroups.

Hence, despite its excellent prognosis, DCIS remains a complex disease process. With regards to patient selection for omission of WBRT a thorough discussion incorporating multiple factors beyond risk stratification alone is warranted which should include an individual patient's risk of relapse using clinical nomograms [66], historic data [67], and more contemporary studies of low-risk patients [60, 64], in addition to placing this risk estimation in context with the patient's co-morbidities, anticipated longevity, preferences of the various management options, and their relative anxiety level pertaining to recurrence versus radiation treatment. It may be that the truly 'low-risk' group, once defined, requires no treatment, a novel concept that is currently being explored in Phase III protocols [68, 69]. Ultimately, these decisions for omission of standard treatments are more likely to impact quality of life measures than breast cancer-related survival outcomes for most 'low-risk' DCIS patients.

7.6   Post-mastectomy Radiation Therapy

The use of PMRT has been widely accepted for patients with four or more positive lymph nodes, but until recently, remained significant controversial in the one to three positive nodes cohort. The more contemporary PMRT trials suggest that for patients with involved axillary nodes who receive systemic chemotherapy after modified radical mastectomy, local-regional relapses, disease-free, and overall survival rates were significantly improved with the receipt of PMRT, though these findings were not uniform across the cohorts. Despite the approximate 10% survival benefit for patients receiving radiation across all of the contemporary PMRT trials [70–72], the 1995 and 2000 Oxford Overviews of PMRT taught us that a statistically significant reduction in the risk of breast cancer-related deaths was counter-balanced by an increase in the risk of non-breast cancer mortality [73, 74]. Based on the analyses of these data, in 2001, a PMRT guideline was published by ASCO initially recommending that the evidence from randomized trials was sufficient to recommend the routine use of PMRT for patients with four or more positive axillary lymph nodes, but remained less clear in patients with 1–3 positive nodes and needed to be individualized based on the totality of risk factors [75]. Subsequently, the NCCN guideline similarly recommended PMRT in patients with four or more positive nodes (category 1), though the panel strengthened the recommendation for the use of PMRT for women with 1–3 positive nodes by adding in a statement to 'strongly consider' PMRT in patients with 1–3 nodes while acknowledging the disagreement in the interpretation of the data in this subgroup (category 2B) [76].

More recently, the most recent update on the Early Breast Cancer Trialists' Collaborative Group (EBCTCG) from 2014, with 22 trials and 8135 patients treated with and without PMRT, has definitely demonstrated that the risk of isolated local failure without simultaneous or subsequent distant failure decreases from 21% without PMRT versus 4.3% with PMRT ($p < 0.001$). This has resulted in a 20-year breast cancer-specific mortality rate of 49.4% versus 41.5% ($p = 0.01$; RR: 0.78). Furthermore, there was no difference in first recurrence or breast cancer mortality when comparing patients with one positive node to those with 2–3 positive nodes [77]. This large body of data, in addition to other published experiences from more contemporary series, has demonstrated that recent local-regional recurrence risk in post-mastectomy setting is well under 5% with the use of modern systemic therapy agents such as anthracyclines, taxanes, targeted therapies, and hormone inhibitors and importantly, that the use of more contemporary radiation techniques is likely diminishing toxicity associated with older radiation techniques. This has led to the recent updating of the ASCO/ASTRO/SSO PMRT guideline, in which the panel unanimously changed the recommendation to include PMRT for patients with 1–3 positive nodes, given that the available evidence now shows that PMRT does, in fact, reduce the risk of local-regional failure (LRF), any recurrence, and breast cancer mortality for patients with T1-2 breast cancer with 1–3 positive axillary nodes. However, they highlight that some subsets of these patients are likely to have such a low absolute risk of LRF that the benefits of PMRT may be outweighed by its potential toxicities. Due to the variations in acceptable thresholds for risk-to-benefit ratios amongst patients and physicians, the panel recommended that the decision for PMRT be made using careful clinical judgement [78].

7.7 Regional Nodal Radiation Therapy

The evolution from ALND to SLNB staging has led to complex clinical considerations for radiation oncologists who must take into account the potential implications of less surgery on radiation treatment fields. In addition, there is a growing body of data to suggest that more comprehensive radiation coverage of regional lymph nodes, both after mastectomy and breast-conserving surgery, may provide a benefit in diminishing the risk of distant metastatic disease in higher-risk patients. While a detailed discussion of the variety of clinical scenarios is beyond the scope of this chapter, considerations of regional nodal radiation have significantly added to the complexity of radiation treatment planning and should be considered for both breast conservation and post-mastectomy patients on a case-by-case basis.

In cases of clinically node-negative, SLN-positive disease treated with adjuvant radiation (with or without systemic treatment), there are now level 1 data demonstrating that long-term survival outcomes are not compromised with the omission of the ALND. Historically, one of the largest studies, conducted at Institute Curie, was a randomized trial which randomized 658 clinically node-negative patients with tumors ≤ 3 cm who all received adjuvant systemic therapy and RT to the breast, to ALND versus axillary RT. There were no differences in either OS or DFS at a follow-up of 15 years, with isolated axillary lymph failures of 1% versus 3%, suggesting that axillary RT to be an excellent alternative to lymphadenectomy [79].

More recently, the ACOSOG Z-0011 trial of clinically node-negative patients with 1-2 positive SLN without gross extra-nodal extension randomized patients to either omission of ALND or completion ALND. Though the results suggested excellent disease-free survival irrespective of whether full ALND was performed, with 5 years local-regional recurrence-free survival of 96.7% (SLND alone) versus 95.7% (ALND) ($p = 0.28$) [80], this study was initially met with some criticism due to its lack of radiation therapy quality assurance and significant variations in the radiation fields delivered. Though the protocol specified radiation be delivered as tangent fields (breast only), a retrospective analysis of a subset of available port films demonstrated that a significant percentage of patients in both arms had protocol violations and was treated with intent to direct the radiation beam to include axillary lymph nodes [81]. Thus, though Z-011 did not provide clarity (for radiation oncologists) as to *which* radiation fields are indicated when ALND is omitted, this study nevertheless confirms the equivalent long-term local-regional relapse rates with or without ALND, with 10-year local-regional recurrence-free survival of 93.2% (ALND arm) and 94.1% (SNB alone arm) ($p = 0.36$) [82], and therefore strongly supports a less aggressive surgical approach than full ALND for clinically node-negative, pathologically node positive patients with 1–2+ sentinel nodes.

In contrast, the EORTC Phase III trial 'After Mapping of the Axilla: Radiotherapy or Surgery?' (AMAROS) provided more clarity for radiation oncologists by specifically demonstrating that axillary RT was equivalent to ALND after positive SNB. This trial addressed the use of radiation to the axilla instead of ALND specifically in tumors ≤ 5 cm with clinically node-negative disease who had 1-2+ sentinel nodes and were randomized to axillary RT or ALND. After a 5-year follow-up period, axillary recurrences remained very low in both groups (ALND, 0.54% vs. axillary RT, 1.03%), with no significant difference in DFS (86.9% vs. 82.7%; $p = 0.18$) or OS (93.3% vs. 92.5%; $p = 0.34$), and axillary RT resulting in less lymphedema than ALND (14% vs. 28%) [83].

Another relevant question and evolving practice pertains to the selection of node-positive (or high risk node-negative) patients (with or without ALND) who may benefit from more comprehensive nodal radiation, to include the undissected portions of level 2 and the level 3 axilla, the supraclavicular and infraclavicular fossae, and the internal mammary chain. It is important to recognize that the patients included in the early PMRT trials that were also included in the Early Breast Cancer Trialists' Collaborative Group PMRT meta-analysis, which resulted in significant reductions in breast cancer-specific mortality in node-positive patients that received PMRT, in fact, had received chest wall *and* regional nodal radiation [77]. Thus, inclusion of regional nodal radiation in higher-risk post-mastectomy patients resulting in long-term disease-specific survival benefits supports the notion that radiation targeting micro-metastatic (local-regional) disease may be preventing distant dissemination and affecting survival outcomes.

Recently, two important phase III trials, the MA.20 study, and the EORTC 22922 trial included patients who had undergone breast-conserving surgery or mastectomy, who were randomized to local-RT (breast or chest wall) alone or both local-RT (breast or chest wall) and extended nodal RT (supraclavicular, infraclavicular, internal mammary and axilla) [84, 85]. Although the two trials differed in various technical aspects of treatment and patient characteristics, both similarly demonstrated that local-regional recurrence-free survival and metastatic breast cancer-free survival were improved with the use of extended RT to include regional nodes (DFS, 82.0% vs. 77.0% and 72.1% vs. 69.1% in the MA.20 and EORTC studies, respectively). Furthermore, aggregate data from these trials suggest a 10-year overall survival benefit (hazard ratio, 0.88; $p = 0.034$) with regional nodal radiation [86].

Nevertheless, the controversy continues because the independent contribution of radiating the internal mammary lymph node chain versus other nodal basins is not discernible in these trials. With respect to radiation fields that intentionally include the IMN chain, (particularly for left-sided breast cancer patients), there are significant concerns for increasing cardiac dose, which, if not carefully delivered, can increase cardiac mortality and hence has the potential to counterbalance the breast cancer-specific survival benefit, as was shown in the earlier Oxford meta-analyses (Fig. 7.4). To date, only one published trial attempted to assess the potential independent benefit of IMN nodal radiation [87]. Patients with node-positive tumors all received postoperative radiation of the chest wall and supraclavicular nodes and were randomly assigned to receive (or not receive) IMN radiation. Unfortunately, despite the reported 10-year overall survival between the two groups demonstrating an absolute benefit of >3% with the use of IMN radiation (62.6% IMN RT vs. 59.3% no-IMN RT), the trial was likely underpowered to statistically detect small differences and this finding was not statistically significant [87].

A more recent population-based analysis of IMN radiation was conducted using a nationwide, Danish prospective population-based cohort that included patients who underwent definitive surgery for unilateral, early-stage node-positive breast cancer where right-sided disease received IMN radiation and left-sided patients were allocated to no-IMN radiation due to its risks of associated radiation-induced heart disease. The primary endpoint, breast cancer-specific survival, was 20.9% versus 23.4% (adjusted HR, 0.85; 95% CI, 0.73 to 0.98; $p = 0.03$), and risk of distant recurrence was 27.4% versus 29.7% (adjusted HR, 0.89; 95% CI, 0.78–1.01; $p = 0.07$) for radiation to IMN versus no-IMN radiation, respectively, with

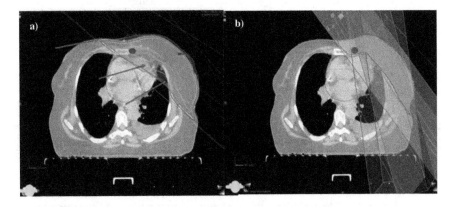

Fig. 7.4 Implications of internal mammary nodal radiation. **a** With tangential techniques that include field-in-field three-dimensional (FIF 3D) treatment, high doses are often delivered to the heart, lung, and contralateral breast (depicted with red arrows). **b** With inverse planned IMRT using multiple planar beams, high doses to heart, lung, and contralateral breast are minimized but entrance and exit of multiple beams result in a higher volume of low-dose radiation to normal tissue

equivalent deaths from ischemic heart disease in both cohorts. These findings led the authors to conclude that IMN radiation increases breast cancer-specific survival outcomes in patients with early-stage, node-positive breast cancer [88].

Hence, the controversy remains as to whether node-positive/high risk node-negative patients treated with regional nodal radiation will result in long-term cardiac morbidity that may jeopardize the potential survival benefits of regional nodal radiation or alternatively, whether these apparent improvements in disease-free survival will ultimately translate into a significant benefit in overall survival with longer follow-up. It is important to recognize, in the context of the techniques utilized in these published studies, that contemporary cardiac avoidance techniques, such as deep inspiration breath hold (as discussed below), which have been shown to significantly diminish the mean heart dose, were not available in the era in which these patients were treated.

In summary, until more mature data become available, the role of regional nodal radiation in low- and high-risk patients is evolving. At this time, it is generally well established that for clinically node-negative patients who have SNB findings of ITCs or micro-metastasis (defined as >0.2–2.0 mm), completion ALND nor regional axillary RT are warranted [89]. However, for patients with multiple macro-metastases on SNB who do not have completion ALND, regional radiation targeting (at a minimum) levels I and II of the axilla are indicated. For patients with 1–2 positive nodes, other factors, (such as age, size of nodal metastasis, estrogen receptor status, tumor biologic subtype, tumor grade, and LVI), should be considered to determine if risk of additional lymph node involvement warrants a completion axillary dissection. Finally, for higher-risk, node-positive patients, particularly those with an otherwise anticipated lengthy longevity, the data suggest additionally targeting the supra-/infraclavicular and the internal mammary chain may improve local-regional control, distant metastasis breast cancer-specific survival, and if meticulously delivered to minimize cardiac exposure, may ultimately portend an overall survival benefit.

7.8   Advances in Radiation Techniques for More Personalized Radiation Delivery

Recent technological advancements have resulted in improvements in the therapeutic ratio of RT, by using three-dimensional, CT-based treatment planning and modulation of the radiation beams to compensate for variations in patients' anatomy. These advances, which have allowed for a more uniform and homogeneous dose across the targeted tissue (i.e., breast and regional nodes), have resulted in diminishing both acute and long-term toxicities to normal breast tissue in addition to minimizing radiation exposure to surrounding structures, such as heart, lung, and unaffected contralateral breast or chest wall, while maintaining tumor control. In selected cases, recent advancements in techniques have allowed for more accelerated treatment delivery approaches such as accelerated partial breast irradiation (aPBI) and hypo-fractionated whole breast radiation (hWBRT), discussed above. In this section, additional advances in external beam radiation therapy technologies will be reviewed.

EBRT is the most widespread and most common method for delivering radiation therapy and most commonly utilizes cobalt machines or linear accelerators (LINACS). Cobalt delivers photon energies of 1.2 and 1.3 MV, which have the ability to adequately penetrate and treat most tumors sites that are not located deep within tissue. Many of the RT trials which originally established the benefits of BCT were delivered using cobalt machines, and with long-term follow-up, the disadvantages of cobalt machines have become more apparent. These include its inherently larger penumbra (less defined beam edge) and inadvertent exposure to normal tissues such as heart, lung, and contralateral breast. The long-term follow-up of patients treated in these early trials has demonstrated the significant consequences of older EBRT techniques. These include higher risks of second malignancy (lung, contralateral breast), cardiovascular disease and cardiac-related deaths specific to left-sided breast cancers [90]. Across North America and Europe, most cobalt machines have been replaced by LINACS, which have the advantages of minimizing personnel exposure, are routinely equipped with a wider variety of beam energies ranging from 4 or 6 MV to 18 or 20 MV photons, in addition to a selection of therapeutic electron beams, which are less penetrating and can be used in combination with photon EBRT to tailor the dose distribution of the beam to the individual patient's body habitus and breast/chest wall contour. Contemporary LINACS also offers automated multi-leaf collimation, intensity modulation capabilities, onboard imaging, and other technological advances all designed to deliver a more precise, conformal dose of radiation.

Traditional breast radiotherapy treatment planning consisted of fluoroscopic simulation to establish treatment fields and a single central axis plane for dose calculations. Given the significant limitations with these 2D-based radiotherapy dose calculations, modern treatment planning techniques now routinely involve use of CT-based, three-dimensional (3D) planning to define the intended target and avoid organs at risk with more accuracy and precision. Increasingly sophisticated algorithms use 3D information to model dose distribution in the radiation field, and modulation of the radiation dose during treatment delivery has greatly improved the ability to ensure adequate target coverage and provide a more homogenous radiation treatment. Several additional technical advances have recently made their way into the clinics and are now considered standard techniques to assist the radiation oncologist to tailor the radiation to the individual patients' body habitus and minimize exposure to normal unaffected tissue.

The vast majority of patients undergoing breast radiation or PMRT will experience some degree of skin toxicity during the standard course of 6-7 weeks of treatment. The severity of skin reactions during and following breast irradiation and the subsequent long-term effects are influenced by both treatment and patient-related factors such as daily fraction size, the total dose delivered, the volume of tissue treated, the type of radiation utilized [91], and the addition of chemotherapy [92]. Additionally, patient-related factors play a large role in the degree of acute and long-term skin changes, for example, breast size, patient age, smoking, risk factors for axillary/arm lymphedema (such as axillary lymph node dissection with large numbers of lymph nodes removed), lymphocele aspiration, history of prior surgical wound infection [93], and most relentlessly, the influence of an individual's genomic constitution, if they are ATM homozygous carriers, which significantly predispose carriers to severe radiation-related complications [94].

Nevertheless, rapid and significant technological advances have allowed for tailoring the radiation beams to the individuals' anatomy. For example, there are now a growing body of data that have consistently demonstrated that more homogeneous dose distributions across the breast volume are directly associated with less acute toxicity such as erythema, skin desquamation, and pain symptoms, as well as long-term toxicity such as palpable and visual fibrosis, retraction of the lumpectomy cavity, development of skin telangiectasia, and ultimate cosmetic outcome [95–97]. Contemporary linear accelerators, which make use of multi-leaf collimation, dynamic wedging, and sub-fields within the original tangent fields to conform the shape and dose of the radiation tangent beams, have allowed for a substantial decrease in the typical inhomogeneities of 125–130% at the central axis seen on breast plans a decade ago to routine breast plans currently with typical inhomogeneity in the <103–107% range.

These improvements in the degree of the dose distribution across treatment plans can be achieved in a number of ways. While two-dimensional techniques were previously utilized to generate standard 'tangent' fields that transect the chest wall medially and laterally, more contemporary planning often will involve forward-planned, field-in-field (FIF-3DCRT) treatment, in which the dose distribution of the tangent fields is examined, and subfields are weighted to optimize the dosimetry. Then, a dose cloud of the 115% isodose curve volume is sequentially generated using multi-leaf collimation onto the medial/lateral tangent fields to block out individual dose clouds (i.e., 115, 110, 107% hot spots) (Fig. 7.5). Typically, 4–6 fields are required to achieve optimization of dose homogeneity, which always include the open medial and lateral fields plus subfields. In addition, the use of higher-energy photons and dynamic wedges can further contour the beam to provide a very conformal and even distribution. Intensity-modulated radiotherapy (IMRT), which is typically planned using treatment planning software, generally delivers more monitor units overall to the patient, uses an inverse planning algorithm to 'sculpt' the dose to the precise volume intended. In the vast majority of cases, the breast inhomogeneity can be reduced to <110% with one of these two methods [98]. Typically, approximately 30% or less of patients can achieve dose homogeneity of ±10% using standard tangents beams only [95]. In patients with hot spots >110%, forward-planned FIF 3D technique should be considered. In cases where FIF 3D techniques with subfields do not achieve the desired homogeneity or often do not spare organs at risk, inverse-planned IMRT can be utilized to generate the beam design, shape, and weighting based on dose specifications, dose constraints, and prioritization of treatment coverage versus the restraints to normal tissue. Multiple beams with sub-beams within them are electronically generated to modulate the dose distribution prioritized to the volume at risk (breast tissue and regional nodes) relative to the organs at risk (heart and lung), and typically can

Fig. 7.5 Whole breast radiation plans: Red depicts hot spots >110%. Top image shows standard tangents, and bottom image utilizes a three-dimensional field-in-field technique to reduce the hot spots, which results in reduced acute and long-term breast toxicities

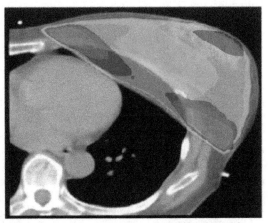

A standard tangential treatment plan treated with wedges. Red isodose depicts hotspots >110%

The same patient planned with a field in field tangential treatment plan, eliminating hotspots >110%

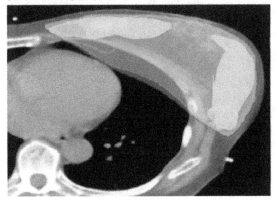

achieve less inhomogeneity in the target tissues, with potentially steeper dose gradients to protect organs at risk. It is important to recognize that inverse planned rotational IMRT, which has the highest scatter dose of any technique, particularly when multiple gantry angles are employed, will result in the patient receiving a larger volume of low-dose radiation, with the potential to increase low-dose exposure to the lung, heart, and contralateral breast tissue, which may have potential concerns for long-term toxicity and secondary malignancies [99].

Lastly, in institutions where proton therapy is available, the use of proton therapy has added to the artillery that has become available, particularly in very challenging cases such as unusual anatomy or prior radiation treatment to an adjacent region. The use of proton therapy shows great promise in reducing cardiac dose. For example, when comparing DIBH versus proton therapy for cardiac avoidance, the mean cardiac dose is shown to be reduced from 1.6 Gy with DIBH to as low as 0.009 Gy with proton therapy [100]. Nevertheless, it is important to remember that achieving such ultra-low doses to the heart (i.e., <2 Gy) has not been shown to have any effects on long-term cardiac morbidity/mortality, so it remains uncertain if protons can provide any additional clinical benefit to justify their expense over the more economical methods available. In summary, while inverse-planned IMRT and proton therapy— can provide excellent homogeneity and normal tissue sparing, the drawbacks of these modalities, including the potential for increased low-dose radiation exposure, increased treatment time, and specifically for proton beam treatment, increased cost, should restrict their use to select cases where acceptable dose constraints are not achievable using other (previously described) technological methods [101–103].

Other relatively simple technological advances have significantly changed the risk vs. benefit profile for breast radiation. For example, breast cancer patients were traditionally positioned in the supine position for treatment planning and delivery. More recently, delivery of EBRT in the prone position has been found to be advantageous in selected patients in moving the majority of breast tissue forward, preventing it from wrapping around the chest wall and abdomen, and elongating its shape, which results in significantly diminishing heart and lung dose and minimizing dose inhomogeneity [104]. When comparing prone and supine positioning, prone positioning has been shown to decrease the volume of heart in 85% of evaluated left-sided breast cancer patients [105] (Fig. 7.6). Selection criteria for use of the prone positioning technique include considerations such as the ability of the patient to comfortably lie on her stomach for extended periods of time, left-sided (vs. right sided) breast cancers, and pendulous or ample breast tissue. Prone positioning is also limited in its utilization for tangential (breast only) treatment, and cannot be used when regional nodes need to be comprehensively included. An additional factor for consideration is tumor bed location, because lumpectomy cavities in close proximity to the chest wall or close to the medial sternum may not receive adequate coverage with the radiation beam. Lastly, bilateral breast radiation is typically a relative contraindication for prone positioning, as it would mandate the patient be repositioned between treatments of each breast, and does not allow for reliable avoidance of mid-sternal overlap.

Another simple technique used to significantly reduce the heart dose is individualization of the treatment field using a heart block, which mandates a review of preoperative imaging to understand the relationship of the tumor to the chest wall. A small lead block is then placed in the radiation beam which functions to block the heart silhouette but must selectively and meticulously place so that critical breast tissue is not blocked. In the appropriate patient, a heart block can significantly decrease the dose to the heart, has been shown to decrease the breast volume coverage by only 2.8%, without any compromise local control [106], and offers a simple method for cardiac avoidance without having to resort to more advanced techniques.

Another more complex cardiac avoidance solution involves a form of respiratory gating termed deep inspiration breath hold (DIBH). This technique takes advantage of the inferior and posterior displacements of the heart when a patient takes a deep inspiration. Two CT scans are performed at the time of CT simulation, one in which

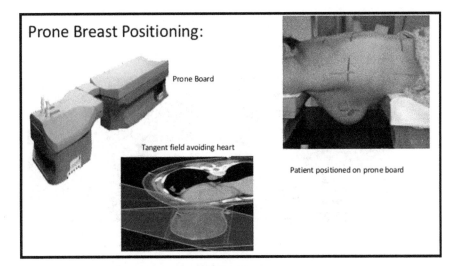

Fig. 7.6 Prone positioning. The board is placed daily onto the treatment machine and positioned with both arms above their heart and affected breast hanging. CT image depicts the breast positioned anteriorly and away from the chest wall, which facilitates cardiac avoidance when placing tangential fields

the patient is supine and breathing freely, the second in which the patient is asked to hold their breath for 20–30 seconds; the position of their chest wall is tracked, and treatment planning is performed off of the breath hold scan. CT-based investigations suggest that heart is completely removed from the radiation field in nearly 50% of patients with a deep inspiration breath hold, and overall, there is an 80% reduction in cardiac volumes [107] (Fig. 7.7). For the actual treatment, the patient is asked to hold their breath for short intervals, the position of their chest wall/breast tissue is tracked using a variety of laser or other tracking devices, and the LINAC machine only delivers the EBRT when the patient is in the breath hold position. Comparisons of techniques suggests that median heart volume receiving greater than 50% of the dose is decreased from 19 to 3% with either inspiratory gating or DIBH [108]. The use of gating or DIBH has notably decreased the cardiac volume and toxicity in the modern era.

7.9 Conclusions

Increasingly, treatment of individual cancers has transitioned from general treatment recommendations based on stage, tumor characteristics, and traditional pathologic features to more advanced methods for categorizing molecular and biologic features of a tumor. Technological advances in radiation therapy are rapidly evolving, and current radiation trials and transitional research are now

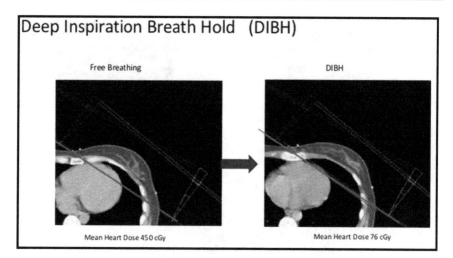

Fig. 7.7 Cardiac avoidance using deep inspiration breath hold. The left scan shows the heart in the tangential field with free breathing. On the right is the DIBH scan which moves the chest wall away from the heart. The treatment is only delivered when the patient is in the maximal breath hold position

started to incorporate a combination of technological specifications in addition to emphasizing methods for identification of tumor characteristics and sub-types that will ultimately result in a more personalized radiotherapy approach. Unlike the field of medical oncology, in which molecular classification and gene assays provide prognostic information, guide treatment decisions, and predict response to systemic treatment, the incorporation of tumor biology into radiation trials remains challenging because the adjuvant radiation setting has no measurable or demonstrable disease activity, and therefore mandates trials designed with significantly longer follow-up time and larger numbers of patients in order to demonstrate small but statistically significant differences (e.g., compared with systemic therapy trials which are often initially explored in the metastatic disease setting). Nevertheless, the field of radiation is rapidly evolving in its own manner and should be delivered using the best available evidence to date, and taking into consideration a variety of additional clinical considerations such as anticipated longevity, quality of life, and patient preferences, and critical technical advancements to account for anatomic considerations to minimize toxicity and maximize the therapeutic ratio. As new data and longer follow-up are reported from prospective randomized trials examining local treatment strategies for breast cancer, clinicians will be, more than ever, challenged with rapidly advancing technology and should exercise caution incorporating them without data establishing their efficacy and safety, since current validated technology demonstrate excellent therapeutic ratios for breast cancer radiation treatment.

References

1. Fisher B, Anderson S, Bryant J, Margolese RG, Deutsch M, Fisher ER et al (2002) Twenty-year follow-up of a randomized trial comparing total mastectomy, lumpectomy, and lumpectomy plus irradiation for the treatment of invasive breast cancer. N Engl J Med 347 (16):1233–1241

2. Litière S, Werutsky G, Fentiman IS, Rutgers E, Christiaens M-R, Van Limbergen E et al (2012) Breast conserving therapy versus mastectomy for stage I-II breast cancer: 20 year follow-up of the EORTC 10801 phase 3 randomised trial. Lancet Oncol 13(4):412–419

3. Poggi MM, Danforth DN, Sciuto LC, Smith SL, Steinberg SM, Liewehr DJ et al (2003) Eighteen-year results in the treatment of early breast carcinoma with mastectomy versus breast conservation therapy: the National Cancer Institute Randomized Trial. Cancer 98 (4):697–702

4. Simone N, Dan T, Shih J, Smith S, Sciuto L, Lita E et al (2012) Twenty-five year results of the national cancer institute randomized breast conservation trial. Breast Cancer Res Treat 132(1):197–203

5. Veronesi U, Cascinelli N, Mariani L, Greco M, Saccozzi R, Luini A et al (2002) Twenty-year follow-up of a randomized study comparing breast-conserving surgery with radical mastectomy for early breast cancer. N Engl J Med 347(16):1227–1232

6. American Cancer Society (2015) Breast cancer facts & figures 2015-2016. American Cancer Society I, Atlanta

7. Gradishar WJ, Hansen NM, Susnik B (2009) Clinical roundtable monograph: a multidisciplinary approach to the use of oncotype DX in clinical practice. Clin Adv Hematol Oncol H&O 7(4):1–7

8. Voduc KD, Cheang MCU, Tyldesley S, Gelmon K, Nielsen TO, Kennecke H (2010) Breast cancer subtypes and the risk of local and regional relapse. J Clin Oncol 28(10):1684–1691

9. Bouganim N, Tsvetkova E, Clemons M, Amir E (2013) Evolution of sites of recurrence after early breast cancer over the last 20 years: implications for patient care and future research. Breast Cancer Res Treat 139(2):603–606

10. Early Breast Cancer Trialists' Collaborative (2011) G. Effect of radiotherapy after breast-conserving surgery on 10-year recurrence and 15-year breast cancer death: meta-analysis of individual patient data for 10, 801 women in 17 randomised trials. Lancet 378(9804):1707–1716

11. Garcia-Etienne CA, Tomatis M, Heil J, Danaei M, Rageth CJ, Marotti L et al (2013) Fluctuating mastectomy rates across time and geography. Ann Surg Oncol 20(7):2114–2116

12. Farrow DC, Hunt WC, Samet JM (1992) Geographic variation in the treatment of localized breast cancer. N Engl J Med 326(17):1097–1101

13. Gabriel G, Barton M, Delaney GP (2015) The effect of travel distance on radiotherapy utilization in NSW and ACT. Radiother Oncol 117(2):386–389

14. Brunt AM, Wheatley D, Yarnold J, Somaiah N, Kelly S, Harnett A et al (2016) Acute skin toxicity associated with a 1-week schedule of whole breast radiotherapy compared with a standard 3-week regimen delivered in the UK FAST-Forward Trial. Radiother Oncol 120(1):114–118

15. Rowe B, Moran MS (2011) Accelerated partial breast irradiation and hypofractionated whole breast radiation. US Oncol Hematol 7(1):31–37

16. Bentzen SM, Agrawal RK, Aird EG, Barrett JM, Barrett-Lee PJ, Bliss JM et al (2008) The UK Standardisation of Breast Radiotherapy (START) Trial A of radiotherapy hypofractionation for treatment of early breast cancer: a randomised trial. Lancet Oncol 9 (4):331–341

17. Whelan TJ, Pignol JP, Levine MN, Julian JA, MacKenzie R, Parpia S et al (2010) Long-term results of hypofractionated radiation therapy for breast cancer. N Engl J Med 362(6): 513–520

18. Haviland JS, Owen JR, Dewar JA, Agrawal RK, Barrett J, Barrett-Lee PJ et al (2013) The UK Standardisation of Breast Radiotherapy (START) trials of radiotherapy hypofractionation for treatment of early breast cancer: 10-year follow-up results of two randomised controlled trials. Lancet Oncol 14(11):1086–1094

19. Group ST, Bentzen SM, Agrawal RK, Aird EG, Barrett JM, Barrett-Lee PJ et al (2008) The UK Standardisation of Breast Radiotherapy (START) Trial B of radiotherapy hypofractionation for treatment of early breast cancer: a randomised trial. Lancet 371 (9618):1098–1107

20. Group FT, Agrawal RK, Alhasso A, Barrett-Lee PJ, Bliss JM, Bliss P et al (2011) First results of the randomised UK FAST Trial of radiotherapy hypofractionation for treatment of early breast cancer (CRUKE/04/015). Radiother Oncol 100(1):93–100

21. Bentzen SM, Agrawal RK, Aird EG, Barrett JM, Barrett-Lee PJ, Bentzen SM et al (2008) The UK Standardisation of Breast Radiotherapy (START) Trial B of radiotherapy hypofractionation for treatment of early breast cancer: a randomised trial. Lancet 371 (9618):1098–1107

22. Smith BD, Bentzen SM, Correa CR, Hahn CA, Hardenbergh PH, Ibbott GS et al (2010) Fractionation for whole breast irradiation: an American Society for Radiation Oncology (ASTRO) evidence-based guideline. Int J Radiat Oncol Biol Phys

23. The Choosing Wisely campaign: American Society for Radiation Oncology 10 Things Physicians and Patients Should Question (n.d.) Retrieved April 7, from http://www.choosingwisely.org/wp-content/uploads/2013/09/ASTRO-5things-List_092013.pdf

24. Vicini FA, Kestin LL, Goldstein NS (2004) Defining the clinical target volume for patients with early-stage breast cancer treated with lumpectomy and accelerated partial breast irradiation: a pathologic analysis. Int J Radiat Oncol Biol Phys 60(3):722–730

25. B Fisher, Anderson S (1994) Conservative surgery for the management of invasive and noninvasive carcinoma of the breast: NSABP trials. National Surgical Adjuvant Breast and Bowel Project. World J Surg 18(1):63–69

26. Clark RM, McCulloch PB, Levine MN, Lipa M, Wilkinson RH, Mahoney LJ et al (1992) Randomized clinical trial to assess the effectiveness of breast irradiation following lumpectomy and axillary disection for node-negative breast cancer. J Natl Cancer Inst 84 (9):683–689

27. Smith TE, Lee D, Turner BC, Carter D, Haffty BG (2000) True recurrence vs. new primary ipsilateral breast tumor relapse: an analysis of clinical and pathologic differences and their implications in natural history, prognoses, and therapeutic management. Int J Radiat Oncol Biol Phys 48(5):1281–1289

28. Liljegren G, Holmberg L, Adami HO, Westman G, Graffman S, Bergh J (1994) Sector resection with or without postoperative radiotherapy for stage I breast cancer: five-year results of a randomized trial. Uppsala-Orebro Breast Cancer Study Group. J Natl Cancer Inst 86(9):717–722

29. Veronesi U, Luini A, Del Vecchio M, Greco M, Galimberti V, Merson M et al (1993) Radiotherapy after breast-preserving surgery in women with localized cancer of the breast. N Engl J Med 328(22):1587–1591

30. Polgár C, Major T, Lövey K et al (2008) Hungarian experience on partial breast irradiation versus whole breast irradiation: 12-year results of a phase II trial and updated results of a randomized study. Brachytherapy 7:91–92[Abstract]

31. Vicini FA, Horwitz EM, Lacerna MD, Dmuchowski CF, Brown DM, White J et al (1997) Long-term outcome with interstitial brachytherapy in the management of patients with early-stage breast cancer treated with breast-conserving therapy. Int J Radiat Oncol Biol Phys 37(4):845–852

32. Vicini FA, Arthur DW (2005) Breast brachytherapy: North American experience. Semin Radiat Oncol 15(2):108–115

33. Khan AJ, Arthur D, Vicini F, Beitsch P, Kuerer H, Goyal S et al (2012) Six-year analysis of treatment-related toxicities in patients treated with accelerated partial breast irradiation on the American Society of Breast Surgeons MammoSite Breast Brachytherapy Registry Trial. Ann Surg Oncol 19(5):1477–1483

34. Vicini F, Beitsch PD, Quiet CA, Keleher AJ, Garcia D, Snider HC Jr et al (2008) Three-year analysis of treatment efficacy, cosmesis, and toxicity by the American Society of Breast Surgeons MammoSite Breast Brachytherapy Registry Trial in patients treated with accelerated partial breast irradiation (APBI). Cancer 112(4):758–766

35. Vicini FA, Beitsch PD, Quiet CA, Keleher A, Garcia D, Snider HC et al (2005) First analysis of patient demographics, technical reproducibility, cosmesis, and early toxicity: results of the American Society of Breast Surgeons MammoSite breast brachytherapy trial. Cancer 104 (6):1138–1148

36. Vicini F, Winter K, Wong J, Pass H, Rabinovitch R, Chafe S et al (2010) Initial Efficacy Results of RTOG 0319: Three-Dimensional Conformal Radiation Therapy (3D-CRT) Confined to the Region of the Lumpectomy Cavity for Stage I/II Breast Carcinoma. Int J Radiat Oncol Biol Phys 77(4):1120–1127

37. Julian TB, JP C, FA V et al (2011) Early toxicity results with 3D conformal external beam (CEBT) from the NSABP B39/RTOG 0413 accelerated partial breast irradiation trial. J Clin Oncol 29:82s (suppl; abstr 1011)

38. Olivotto IA, Whelan TJ, Parpia S, Kim D-H, Berrang T, Truong PT et al (2013) Interim cosmetic and toxicity results from RAPID: a randomized trial of accelerated partial breast irradiation using three-dimensional conformal external beam radiation therapy. J Clin Oncol 31(32):4038–4045

39. Hepel JT, Tokita M, MacAusland SG, Evans SB, Hiatt JR, Price LL et al (2009) Toxicity of three-dimensional conformal radiotherapy for accelerated partial breast irradiation. Int J Radiat Oncol Biol Phys 75(5):1290–1296

40. Jagsi R, Ben-David MA, Moran JM, Marsh RB, Griffith KA, Hayman JA et al (2010) Unacceptable cosmesis in a protocol investigating intensity-modulated radiotherapy with active breathing control for accelerated partial-breast irradiation. Int J Radiat Oncol Biol Phys 76(1):71–78

41. Moran MS, Truong PT (2014) Intraoperative accelerated partial breast irradiation: caution still warranted. Int J Radiat Oncol Biol Phys 89(3):496–498

42. Veronesi U, Orecchia R, Maisonneuve P, Viale G, Rotmensz N, Sangalli C et al (2013) Intraoperative radiotherapy versus external radiotherapy for early breast cancer (ELIOT): a randomised controlled equivalence trial. Lancet Oncol 14(13):1269–1277

43. Veronesi U, Orecchia R, Luini A, Galimberti V, Zurrida S, Intra M et al (2010) Intraoperative radiotherapy during breast conserving surgery: a study on 1,822 cases treated with electrons. Breast Cancer Res Treat 124(1):141–151

44. Vaidya JS, Wenz F, Bulsara M, Tobias JS, Joseph DJ, Keshtgar M et al (2014) Risk-adapted targeted intraoperative radiotherapy versus whole-breast radiotherapy for breast cancer: 5-year results for local control and overall survival from the TARGIT-A randomised trial. Lancet 383(9917):603–613

45. Smith BD, Arthur DW, Buchholz TA, Haffty BG, Hahn CA, Hardenbergh PH et al (2009) Accelerated partial breast irradiation consensus statement from the American Society for Radiation Oncology (ASTRO). J Am Coll Surg 209(2):269–277

46. Correa C, Harris EE, Leonardi MC, Smith BD, Taghian AG, Thompson AM et al (2016) Accelerated partial breast irradiation: executive summary for the update of an ASTRO evidence-based consensus statement. Pract Radiat Oncol

47. Moran MS, Schnitt SJ, Giuliano AE, Harris JR, Khan SA, Horton J et al (2014) Society of surgical oncology-American society for radiation oncology consensus guideline on margins for breast-conserving surgery with whole-breast irradiation in stages I and II invasive breast cancer. J Clin Oncol

48. Hughes KS, Schnaper LA, Berry D, Cirrincione C, McCormick B, Shank B et al (2004) Lumpectomy plus tamoxifen with or without irradiation in women 70 years of age or older with early breast cancer. N Engl J Med 351(10):971–977
49. Kunkler IH, Williams LJ, Jack WJL, Cameron DA, Dixon JM (2015) Breast-conserving surgery with or without irradiation in women aged 65 years or older with early breast cancer (PRIME II): a randomised controlled trial. Lancet Oncol 16(3):266–273
50. Hughes KS, Schnaper LA, Bellon JR, Cirrincione CT, Berry DA, McCormick B et al (2013) Lumpectomy plus tamoxifen with or without irradiation in women age 70 years or older with early breast cancer: long-term follow-up of CALGB 9343. J Clin Oncol 31(19):2382–2387
51. Blamey RW, Bates T, Chetty U, Duffy SW, Ellis IO, George D et al (2013) Radiotherapy or tamoxifen after conserving surgery for breast cancers of excellent prognosis: British Association of Surgical Oncology (BASO) II trial. Eur J Cancer 49(10):2294–2302
52. Gradishar WJ, Anderson BO, Balassanian R, Blair SL, Burstein HJ, Cyr A et al (2016) Invasive breast cancer version 1.2016, NCCN clinical practice guidelines in oncology. J Natl Compr Canc Netw 14(3):324–354
53. Palta M, Palta P, Bhavsar NA, Horton JK, Blitzblau RC (2015) The use of adjuvant radiotherapy in elderly patients with early-stage breast cancer: changes in practice patterns after publication of Cancer and Leukemia Group B 9343. Cancer 121(2):188–193
54. Morrow M, Van Zee KJ, Solin LJ, Houssami N, Chavez-MacGregor M, Harris JR et al (2016) Society of surgical oncology-American society for radiation oncology-American Society of clinical oncology consensus guideline on margins for breast-conserving surgery with whole-breast irradiation in ductal carcinoma in situ. Ann Surg Oncol
55. Wärnberg F, Garmo H, Emdin S, Hedberg V, Adwall L, Sandelin K et al (2014) Effect of radiotherapy after breast-conserving surgery for ductal carcinoma in situ: 20 years follow-up in the randomized SweDCIS trial. J Clin Oncol 32(32):3613–3618
56. Donker M, Litière S, Werutsky G, Julien J-P, Fentiman IS, Agresti R et al (2013) Breast-conserving treatment with or without radiotherapy in ductal carcinoma in situ: 15-year recurrence rates and outcome after a recurrence, from the EORTC 10853 randomized phase III trial. J Clin Oncol
57. Cuzick J, Sestak I, Pinder SE, Ellis IO, Forsyth S, Bundred NJ et al (2011) Effect of tamoxifen and radiotherapy in women with locally excised ductal carcinoma in situ: long-term results from the UK/ANZ DCIS trial. Lancet Oncol 12(1):21–29
58. Wapnir I, Dignam J, Fisher B, Mamounas E, Anderson S, Julian T et al (2011) Long-term outcomes of invasive ipsilateral breast tumor recurrences after lumpectomy in NSABP B-17 and B-24 randomized clinical trials for DCIS. J Natl Cancer Inst 103(6):478–488
59. Moran MS (2015) Ductal Carcinoma in situ and relevant endpoints for omission of standard treatments: are we there yet? ASCO Post 2015;Dec 25, 2015. http://www.ascopost.com/issues/december-25-2015/ductal-carcinoma-in-situ-and-relevant-endpoints-for-omission-of-standard-treatments-are-we-there-yet/
60. McCormick B, Winter K, Hudis C, Kuerer HM, Rakovitch E, Smith BL et al (2015) RTOG 9804: a prospective randomized trial for good-risk ductal carcinoma in situ comparing radiotherapy with observation. J Clin Oncol
61. Wong JS, Kaelin CM, Troyan SL, Gadd MA, Gelman R, Lester SC et al (2006) Prospective study of wide excision alone for ductal carcinoma in situ of the breast. J Clin Oncol 24(7):1031–1036
62. Wong JS, Chen YH, Gadd MA, Gelman R, Lester SC, Schnitt SJ et al (2014) Eight-year update of a prospective study of wide excision alone for small low- or intermediate-grade ductal carcinoma in situ (DCIS). Breast Cancer Res Treat 143(2):343–350
63. Hughes LL, Wang M, Page DL, Gray R, Solin LJ, Davidson NE et al (2009) Local excision alone without irradiation for ductal carcinoma in situ of the breast: a trial of the Eastern Cooperative Oncology Group. J Clin Oncol 27(32):5319–5324

64. Solin LJ, Gray R, Hughes LL, Wood WC, Lowen MA, Badve SS et al (2015) Surgical excision without radiation for ductal carcinoma in situ of the breast: 12-year results from the ECOG-ACRIN E5194 study. J Clin Oncol

65. Rakovitch E, Nofech-Mozes S, Hanna W, Baehner F, Saskin R, Butler S et al (2015) A population-based validation study of the DCIS Score predicting recurrence risk in individuals treated by breast-conserving surgery alone. Breast Cancer Res Treat 152 (2):389–398

66. Rudloff U, Jacks LM, Goldberg JI, Wynveen CA, Brogi E, Patil S et al (2010) Nomogram for predicting the risk of local recurrence after breast-conserving surgery for ductal carcinoma in situ. J Clin Oncol 28(23):3762–3769

67. EBCTCG (2010) Overview of the randomized trials of radiotherapy in ductal carcinoma in situ of the breast. JNCI Monogr 2010(41):162–177

68. Elshof LE, Tryfonidis K, Slaets L, van Leeuwen-Stok AE, Skinner VP, Dif N et al (2015) Feasibility of a prospective, randomised, open-label, international multicentre, phase III, non-inferiority trial to assess the safety of active surveillance for low risk ductal carcinoma in situ—the LORD study. Eur J Cancer 51(12):1497–1510

69. Francis A, Thomas J, Fallowfield L, Wallis M, Bartlett JMS, Brookes C et al (2015) Addressing overtreatment of screen detected DCIS; the LORIS trial. Eur J Cancer 51 (16):2296–2303

70. Ragaz J, Jackson SM, Le N, Plenderleith IH, Spinelli JJ, Basco VE et al (1997) Adjuvant radiotherapy and chemotherapy in node-positive premenopausal women with breast cancer. N Engl J Med 337(14):956–962

71. Overgaard M, Hansen PS, Overgaard J, Rose C, Andersson M, Bach F et al (1997) Postoperative radiotherapy in high-risk premenopausal women with breast cancer who receive adjuvant chemotherapy. Danish Breast Cancer Cooperative Group 82b Trial. N Engl J Med 337(14):949–955

72. Overgaard M, Jensen MB, Overgaard J, Hansen PS, Rose C, Andersson M et al (1999) Postoperative radiotherapy in high-risk postmenopausal breast-cancer patients given adjuvant tamoxifen: Danish Breast Cancer Cooperative Group DBCG 82c randomised trial. Lancet 353(9165):1641–1648

73. Group EBCTC (1995) Effects of radiotherapy and surgery in early breast cancer—an overview of the randomized trials. N Engl J Med 333(22):1444–1456

74. Early Breast Cancer Trialists' Collaborative (2000) G. Favourable and unfavourable effects on long-term survival of radiotherapy for early breast cancer: an overview of the randomised trials. Lancet 355(9217):1757–1770

75. Recht A, Edge SB, Solin LJ, Robinson DS, Estabrook A, Fine RE et al (2001) Postmastectomy radiotherapy: clinical practice guidelines of the american society of clinical oncology. J Clin Oncol 19(5):1539–1569

76. Carlson RW, McCormick B (2005) Update: NCCN breast cancer clinical practice guidelines. J Natl Compr Cancer Netw JNCCN 3(Suppl 1):S7–S11

77. EBCTCG (2014) Effect of radiotherapy after mastectomy and axillary surgery on 10-year recurrence and 20-year breast cancer mortality: meta-analysis of individual patient data for 8135 women in 22 randomised trials. Lancet

78. Recht A, Comen EA, Fine RE, Fleming GF, Hardenbergh PH, Ho AY et al (2016) Postmastectomy radiotherapy: an american society of clinical oncology, American Society for Radiation Oncology, and Society of Surgical Oncology Focused Guideline Update. J Clin Oncol

79. Louis-Sylvestre C, Clough K, Asselain B, Vilcoq JR, Salmon RJ, Fß Campana et al (2004) Axillary treatment in conservative management of operable breast cancer: dissection or radiotherapy? results of a randomized study with 15 years of follow-up. J Clin Oncol 22(1):97–101

80. Giuliano AE, Hunt KK, Ballman KV, Beitsch PD, Whitworth PW, Blumencranz PW et al (2011) Axillary dissection vs no axillary dissection in women with invasive breast cancer and sentinel node metastasis: a randomized clinical trial. JAMA 305(6):569–575

81. Jagsi R, Chadha M, Moni J, Ballman K, Laurie F, Buchholz TA et al (2014) Radiation field design in the ACOSOG Z0011 (Alliance) trial. J Clin Oncol

82. Giuliano Aea (2016) Ten-year survival results of ACOSOG Z0011: a randomized trial of axillary node dissection in women with clinical T1-2 N0 M0 breast cancer who have a positive sentinel node (Alliance). J Clin Oncol 34 (suppl; abstr 1007)

83. Donker M, van Tienhoven G, Straver ME, Meijnen P, van de Velde CJ, Mansel RE et al (2014) Radiotherapy or surgery of the axilla after a positive sentinel node in breast cancer (EORTC 10981-22023 AMAROS): a randomised, multicentre, open-label, phase 3 non-inferiority trial. Lancet Oncol 15(12):1303–1310

84. Poortmans PM, Collette S, Kirkove C, Van Limbergen E, Budach V, Struikmans H et al (2015) Internal mammary and medial supraclavicular irradiation in breast cancer. N Engl J Med 373(4):317–327

85. Whelan TJ, Olivotto IA, Parulekar WR, Ackerman I, Chua BH, Nabid A et al (2015) Regional nodal irradiation in early-stage breast cancer. N Engl J Med 373(4):307–316

86. Budach W, Bolke E, Kammers K, Gerber PA, Nestle-Kramling C, Matuschek C (2015) Adjuvant radiation therapy of regional lymph nodes in breast cancer—a meta-analysis of randomized trials—an update. Radiat Oncol 10:258

87. Hennequin C, Bossard N, Servagi-Vernat S, Maingon P, Dubois JB, Datchary J et al (2013) Ten-year survival results of a randomized trial of irradiation of internal mammary nodes after mastectomy. Int J Radiat Oncol Biol Phys 86(5):860–866

88. Thorsen LB, Offersen BV, Dano H, Berg M, Jensen I, Pedersen AN et al (2016) DBCG-IMN: a population-based cohort study on the effect of internal mammary node irradiation in early node-positive breast cancer. J Clin Oncol 34(4):314–320

89. Galimberti V, Cole BF, Zurrida S, Viale G, Luini A, Veronesi P et al (2013) IBCSG 23-01 randomised controlled trial comparing axillary dissection versus no axillary dissection in patients with sentinel node micrometastases. Lancet Oncol 14(4):297–305

90. Clarke M, Collins R, Darby S, Davies C, Elphinstone P, Evans V et al (2005) Effects of radiotherapy and of differences in the extent of surgery for early breast cancer on local recurrence and 15-year survival: an overview of the randomised trials. Lancet 366 (9503):2087–2106

91. Hall EJ, Giaccia AJ (2012) Radiobiology for the radiologist (edition 7E, 2012). 6th edn. Philadelphia: Lippincott Williams & Wilkins. ix, 546 pp

92. Bentzen SM, Turesson I, Thames HD (1990) Fractionation sensitivity and latency of telangiectasia after postmastectomy radiotherapy: a graded-response analysis. Radiother Oncol 18:95–106

93. Porock D, Kristjanson L, Nikoletti S, Cameron F, Pedler P (1998) Predicting the severity of radiation skin reactions in women with breast cancer. Oncol Nurs Forum 25(6):1019–1029

94. Iannuzzi CM, Atencio DP, Green S, Stock RG, Rosenstein BS (2002) ATM mutations in female breast cancer patients predict for an increase in radiation-induced late effects. Int J Radiat Oncol Biol Phys 52(3):606–613

95. Barnett GC, Wilkinson JS, Moody AM, Wilson CB, Twyman N, Wishart GC et al (2011) The Cambridge breast intensity-modulated radiotherapy trial: patient- and treatment-related factors that influence late toxicity. Clin Oncol 23(10):662–673

96. Pignol JP, Olivotto I, Rakovitch E, Gardner S, Sixel K, Beckham W et al (2008) A multicenter randomized trial of breast intensity-modulated radiation therapy to reduce acute radiation dermatitis. J Clin Oncol 26(13):2085–2092

97. Mukesh MB, Barnett GC, Wilkinson JS, Moody AM, Wilson C, Dorling L et al (2013) Randomized controlled trial of intensity-modulated radiotherapy for early breast cancer: 5-year results confirm superior overall cosmesis. J Clin Oncol 31(36):4488–4495

98. Moran MS, Haffty BG (2009) Radiation techniques and toxicities for locally advanced breast cancer. Semin Radiat Oncol 19(4):244–255

99. Hall EJ, Wuu CS (2003) Radiation-induced second cancers: the impact of 3D-CRT and IMRT. Int J Radiat Oncol Biol Phys 56(1):83–88

100. Lin LL, Vennarini S, Dimofte A, Ravanelli D, Shillington K, Batra S et al (2015) Proton beam versus photon beam dose to the heart and left anterior descending artery for left-sided breast cancer. Acta Oncol 54(7):1032–1039

101. Smith BD, Pan IW, Shih YC, Smith GL, Harris JR, Punglia R et al (2011) Adoption of intensity-modulated radiation therapy for breast cancer in the United States. J Natl Cancer Inst 103(10):798–809

102. Kurtz JM, Spitalier JM (1990) Local recurrence after breast-conserving surgery and radiotherapy: what have we learned? Int J Radiat Oncol Biol Phys 19(4):1087–1089

103. Cammarota F, Giugliano FM, Iadanza L, Cutillo L, Muto M, Toledo D et al (2014) Hypofractionated breast cancer radiotherapy. Helical tomotherapy in supine position or classic 3D-conformal radiotherapy in prone position: which is better? Anticancer Res 34 (3):1233–1238

104. Goodman KA, Hong L, Wagman R, Hunt MA, McCormick B (2004) Dosimetric analysis of a simplified intensity modulation technique for prone breast radiotherapy. Int J Radiat Oncol Biol Phys 60(1):95–102

105. Formenti SC, DeWyngaert JK, Jozsef G, Goldberg JD (2012) Prone vs supine positioning for breast cancer radiotherapy. JAMA 308(9):861–863

106. Raj KA, Evans ES, Prosnitz RG, Quaranta BP, Hardenbergh PH, Hollis DR et al (2006) Is there an increased risk of local recurrence under the heart block in patients with left-sided breast cancer? Cancer J 12(4):309–317

107. Lu HM, Cash E, Chen MH, Chin L, Manning WJ, Harris J et al (2000) Reduction of cardiac volume in left-breast treatment fields by respiratory maneuvers: a CT study. Int J Radiat Oncol Biol Phys 47(4):895–904

108. Korreman SS, Pedersen AN, Nottrup TJ, Specht L, Nystrom H (2005) Breathing adapted radiotherapy for breast cancer: comparison of free breathing gating with the breath-hold technique. Radiother Oncol J Euro Soc Ther Radiol Oncol 76(3):311–318

Multi-gene Panel Testing in Breast Cancer Management

8

Christos Fountzilas and Virginia G. Kaklamani

Contents

Abstract

Hereditary predisposition accounts for approximately 10% of all breast cancers and is mostly associated with germline mutations in high-penetrance genes encoding for proteins participating in DNA repair through homologous recombination (*BRCA1* and *BRCA2*). With the advent of massive parallel next-generation DNA sequencing, simultaneous analysis of multiple genes with a short turnaround time and at a low cost has become possible. The clinical validity and utility of multi-gene panel testing is getting better characterized as more data on the significance of moderate-penetrance genes are collected from large, cancer genetic testing studies. In this chapter, we attempt to provide a general guide for interpretation of panel gene testing in breast cancer and use of the information obtained for clinical decision-making.

C. Fountzilas · V. G. Kaklamani (✉)
Cancer Therapy and Research Center, University of Texas Health Science Center San Antonio, 7979 Wurzbach Road, San Antonio, TX 78229, USA
e-mail: kaklamani@uthscsa.edu

© Springer International Publishing AG 2018
W. J. Gradishar (ed.), *Optimizing Breast Cancer Management*, Cancer Treatment and Research 173, https://doi.org/10.1007/978-3-319-70197-4_8

Keywords
Hereditary breast cancer syndrome · BRCA1/2 · Deleterious mutations
Gene panel testing · Penetrance · Prevention

8.1   Introduction

Hereditary predisposition is found in approximately 10% of all breast cancer cases [1]. Most hereditary breast cancer cases are related to germline mutations in high-penetrance genes like *BRCA1, BRCA2, PTEN, CDH1, STK11,* and *P53* [2] and follow an autosomal dominant pattern of inheritance.

The genes most commonly involved in hereditary breast (and ovarian) cancer syndromes are *BRCA1* (located on chromosome 17q21) and *BRCA2* (located on chromosome 13q12.3) and encode for proteins that participate in the DNA repair process through homologous recombination [3, 4]. The overall prevalence of deleterious *BRCA1* and *BRCA2* mutations ranges between 1/400 and 1/800 [5, 6] in the general population; the frequency depends on the patient's age and ethnic group; the frequency decreases with age and is higher in patients of Ashkenazi Jewish ancestry [6–8]. More than 1000 mutations for each gene have been discovered; mostly frameshift deletions, insertions, and nonsense mutations that result in a truncated, dysfunctional protein [3]. The frequency of each mutation varies, but founder mutations have been found, for example, *BRCA1* mutations 185delAG and 5382InsC and *BRCA2* mutation 6174delT are recurring genetic alterations in Ashkenazi Jews [9–11]. The lifetime risk of developing breast cancer in *BRCA1/2* carriers ranges between 60 and 70% and 50 and 75%, respectively; the risk of ovarian cancer is 40–60% and 18–65%, respectively [12–15]. Two-thirds of the breast cancer cases associated with germline *BRCA1* mutations have a triple-negative phenotype, while this occurs only in 16% of germline *BRCA2* mutations cases [16]. Patients with *BRCA1/2* germline mutations are also at increased risk for other malignancies such as ovarian cancer, pancreatic cancer, prostate cancer, and melanoma [2].

Other very rare, high-penetrance genes include *P53* (Li-Fraumeni syndrome) [17], *PTEN* (Cowden syndrome) [18], *STK11* (Peutz–Jeghers syndrome) [19], and *CDH1* (hereditary diffuse gastric cancer syndrome). The individual incidence for each of those syndromes is as low as 1 in 280,000 live births [2]. The risk of any invasive cancer in patients with the Li-Fraumeni syndrome is 50% by the age of 30 and 90% by the age of 70 [20]; sarcoma, breast, adrenocortical, and brain cancer as well as leukemia predominate in the clinical picture, but virtually any malignancy is possible [2]. Patients with Cowden syndrome have up to 50% lifetime risk of developing breast cancer as well as 10% risk of thyroid cancer; skin lesions and intestinal hamartomas are commonly found [2]. Gastrointestinal malignancies as a group are the most common cancers in patients with the Peutz–Jeghers syndrome, and the risk of breast cancer by age 65 is 54% [2]. Patients with hereditary diffuse gastric cancer syndrome had a 39% risk of lobular breast carcinoma and more than 67% risk for diffuse gastric cancer [21].

Apart from mutations in high-penetrance genes, mutations in intermediate (relative risk 2–4)- and low (relative risk < 2)-penetrance genes have been identified [22]. In general, mutations in moderate-penetrance genes like *CHEK2* and *ATM,* are more commonly found in women with breast cancer, but the relative increase in the risk of breast cancer is low (relative risk < 3) [23]. The frequency of mutations in high-penetrance genes is lower, but the attributable risk is higher [22]. Mutations in genes so far identified can explain approximately 20% of familiar breast cancer risk [24].

Identification of patients and families with genetic alterations conferring an increased risk for breast and other malignancies is of paramount importance as it can have implications in management of their disease and prevention strategies, respectively. For example, risk-reducing oophorectomy can decrease all cause, breast and ovarian cancer mortality in *BRCA1* and *2* carriers [25]. Also, the use of MRI for breast cancer screening can help detect breast cancers at an earlier stage [26, 27].

8.2 Multi-gene Panel Testing Through Next-Generation Sequencing (NGS)

Nowadays, the ability to detect multiple germline and somatic mutations at a short period of time and with a reasonable cost has greatly improved with the advent of massive parallel next-generation DNA sequencing that has largely replaced Sanger sequencing. After the invalidation of the *BRCA1/2* patents by the US Supreme Court [28], there has been a plethora of companies offering genetic testing, each panel covering more than 100 genes.

We should approach multi-gene panel testing for cancer susceptibility the same way any diagnostic test is evaluated, examining its analytic validity (e.g., accuracy in detecting the presence or absence of a specific mutation), clinical validity (e.g., ability to segregate patients in groups of clearly defined cancer risk), and more importantly clinical utility (e.g., ability to guide decision-making for the individual patient or person tested) as well as its ethical, legal, and social implications [29].

8.2.1 Analytic Validity

Multi-gene panel testing using NGS technologies has a high rate of analytic concordance (approximating 100%) with more traditional sequencing methods such as Sanger sequencing or multiplex ligation-dependent probe amplification (MLPA) [30], allowing us to use results for clinical decision-making.

8.2.2 Clinical Validity

Rather than a dichotomous positive or negative answer regarding the presence or not of a genetic predisposition for breast cancer, genetic testing results provide a range of hereditary risk of breast (or other) cancer risk. Individuals tested may be found to have one of the well-defined hereditary cancer syndromes, or they may have a genetic alteration offering a risk comparable to other benign or premalignant diseases of the breast like atypical ductal hyperplasia (ADH) or lobular carcinoma in situ (LCIS) or have a risk that cannot be defined as approximately 50% of individuals with familiar breast cancer syndrome tested have a genetically unexplained predisposition [31].

The majority of genes associated with an increased risk of breast cancer are coding for proteins participating in the DNA repair process [32]. Most pathogenic variants of breast cancer predisposition genes contain nonsense mutations and frameshift short insertions or deletions producing a truncated, nonfunctional protein [32].

Not all *BRCA1/2* gene variants confer an increased genetic risk for breast cancer. The International Agency for Cancer Research (IARC) 5-tier system classifies variants based on the posterior probability of pathogenicity using a multifactorial likelihood model (Table 8.1) and is intended to help differentiate between high-risk (equivalent to protein-truncating variant) and low- or no-risk variants [33]. The Evidence-based Network for the Interpretation of Germline Mutant Alleles (ENIGMA) consortium variant classification criteria incorporate the IARC classification [33], the ENIGMA system for interpretation of possible spliceogenic variants and splicing alterations [34] and general elements of gene variant classification developed by InSIGHT and the American College of Genetics and Genomics (ACMG) (Table 8.2) [35, 36]. A multifactorial model can incorporate epidemiological/observational/clinical parameters (such as co-segregation of variants in pedigrees, personal and family history of cancer, tumor characteristics and histological grade, and co-occurrence with known pathogenic mutations), in silico analytical data (amino acid conservation within species, changes in physicochemical properties of the amino acid), and splicing predictions as well as functional data at the protein level [37–46]. Variants are classified as pathogenic if their probability is >99%, likely pathogenic if their probability is 95–99%, uncertain (variant of uncertain significance—VUS) if their probability is 5–94%, likely not pathogenic if their probability is 1–4.9%, and not pathogenic if the probability of pathogenicity is >1%. Contrary to pathogenic variants, VUSs are in most cases missense, in-frame

Table 8.1 International Agency for Cancer Research (IARC) 5-tiered classification system [33]

Class	Probability of pathogenicity (%)
5. 5: Pathogenic	>99
4: Likely pathogenic	95–99
3: Uncertain	5–94.9
2: Likely not pathogenic or of little clinical significance	0.1–4.9
1: Not pathogenic or of no clinical significance	<0.1

Table 8.2 Evidence-based Network for the Interpretation of Germline Mutant Alleles (ENIGMA) consortium variant classification criteria [33–36]

Class	Criterion
Class 5: pathogenic	• Posterior probability of pathogenicity > 0.99 from multifactorial likelihood analysis • Coding sequence variant encoding a premature termination codon i.e., nonsense/frameshift predicted to disrupt expression of clinically important functional domain(s) • The variant allele produces only transcripts that lead to a premature stop codon, or in-frame deletion predicted to disrupt clinically important domains, as determined by RNA assays on patient germline tissue that assess allele-specific transcript expression • Copy number deletion removing exon(s) spanning clinically important functional domain(s) or proven to result in a frameshift alteration predicted to interrupt expression of clinically important functional domain(s) • Copy number duplication proven to result in frameshift alteration predicted to interrupt expression of clinically important functional domain(s)
Class 4: likely pathogenic	• Posterior probability of pathogenicity 0.95–0.99 from multifactorial likelihood analysis • Variant at IVS $\pm$ 1 or IVS $\pm$ 2 or G > non-G at last base of exon when adjacent intronic sequence is not GTRRGT but is untested for splicing aberrations using RNA assays on patient blood that assess allele-specific transcript expression and is not predicted or known to lead to naturally occurring in-frame RNA isoforms that may rescue gene functionality • A variant that encodes the same amino acid change as a previously established class 5 pathogenic missense variant with a different underlying nucleotide change is located in a known clinically important functional protein domain, with no evidence of mRNA aberration (splicing or expression) from in vitro mRNA assays on patient RNA, and the variant is absent from outbred control reference groups • A small in-frame deletion variant that removes a codon for which a missense substitution class 5 variant has been described is located in a known clinically important functional protein domain and is absent from outbred control reference groups
Class 3: uncertain	• Posterior probability of pathogenicity 0.05–0.949 from multifactorial likelihood analysis • Insufficient evidence to classify variant • Variant located at specific positions, unless proven to fall in another class based on additional evidence • Variant with conflicting evidence for pathogenicity

(continued)

Table 8.2 (continued)

Class	Criterion
Class 2: Likely not pathogenic or of little clinical significance	• Posterior probability of pathogenicity 0.001–0.049 from multifactorial likelihood analysis • Exonic variant that encodes the same amino acid change as a previously established class 1 not pathogenic missense variant with a different underlying nucleotide change, and for which there is no evidence of mRNA aberration from in vitro mRNA assays
Class 1: not pathogenic or of no clinical significance	• Posterior probability of pathogenicity <0.001 from multifactorial likelihood analysis • Variant with reported frequency $\geq 1\%$ in large outbred control reference groups • Exonic variant encoding missense or small in-frame alteration at a position that is not evolutionary conserved or synonymous substitution or intronic variant • there is bioinformatic prediction of an effect on splicing • And there is no associated variant-specific mRNA aberration in lab assays • Or the variant co-occurs in trans with a known pathogenic sequence variant in the same gene in an individual who has no obvious additional clinical phenotype other than BRCA-associated cancer • Exonic variant encoding missense or small in-frame alteration at a position that is not evolutionary conserved or synonymous substitution or intronic variant • there is no bioinformatic prediction of altered splicing • the variant co-occurs in trans with a known pathogenic sequence variant in the same gene in an individual who has no obvious additional clinical phenotype other than BRCA-associated cancer

deletions/insertions, and intronic mutations [32]; most pathogenic *BRCA1* missense mutations are located in domains crucial for the protein's DNA repair activity (RING and BRCT) while most pathogenic missense *BRCA2* mutations in the DNA binding domain [31, 47], but just the presence of a missense mutation within a critical region of the gene does not confer increased risk. For example, the missense mutation p.Arg1699Gln (R1699Q) in the BRCT domain of *BRCA1* increases the risk compared to general population but less so compared to standard *BRCA1* penetrance (24% vs. 65% by age 70) [14, 48]. Even for truncating variants though, the risk of breast cancer is not uniform, depending on the location of the alteration within the gene [49]. The truncated variant *BRCA2* rs11571833 confers only a modestly increased risk (odds ratio 1.39; 95% CI: 1.13–1.71, $P = 0.0016$) [50]. Further, the risk of breast cancer among *BRCA* carriers appears also to be modified by the presence single nucleotide polymorphisms (SNPs) in low-penetrance genes [51, 52].

In specific mutation-negative relatives of known *BRCA* mutation carriers, the risk of breast cancer does not appear statistically significantly increased compared to the general population with risk ratios ranging from 0.39 to 2.9 in individual prospective and population-based studies [53–56].

In cases of Li-Fraumeni syndrome, both p53 protein-truncating and missense variants appear to confer an increased risk [57, 58]. The standardized incidence ratio (SIR) for breast cancer is 105.1 (95% CI 55.9–179.8) in p53 mutation carriers [58] and 25.4 (95% CI 19.8–32.0) in *PTEN* mutation carriers [59]. The relative risk for breast cancer (especially the lobular carcinoma subtype) is 6.6—slightly above the threshold for high-penetrance characterization—in patients with truncating variants of *CDH1* [21] and 6 in patients with Peutz–Jeghers syndrome [60].

PALB2 (partner and localizer of *BRCA2*) is a gene encoding for a BRCA1 and 2-interacting protein essential for their function. Whether *PALB2* is a high-penetrance gene has been a matter of debate. Several studies estimate the risk for heterozygotes as being less than 4 [61, 62], while variant c.1592delT was associated with a 14-fold (95% CI, 6.6–31.2) [63] and variant c.3113G > A with a 30-fold (95% CI 7.5–120) increased risk for breast cancer in a Finnish and Australian population respectively [64]. In the multinational study by Antoniou et al., *PALB2* mutation carriers had a relative risk of 9.47 (95% CI, 7.16–12.57) for breast cancer [65]. The most common mutations detected were c.1592del and c.3113G > A. Couch et al. [23] reported at the 2016 San Antonio Breast Cancer Symposium the results of germline testing in almost 40,000 breast cancer patients in a nationwide hereditary cancer genetic testing program. The majority of the patients were Caucasian between the ages of 40 and 65. *PALB2* mutations were detected in 0.40% of the population. In this study, carriers of pathogenic *PALB2* had a sevenfold increase in the odds for breast cancer, a finding that likely confirms *PALB2* as a high-penetrance gene.

ATM gene (ataxia-telangiectasia mutated) encodes for a DNA damage signal protein and is considered a moderate-penetrance gene. In the study by Couch et al., the odds ratio for development of breast cancer was 2.83 (CI 95% 2.23–3.64) [23]. As in the case of high-penetrance genes, missense mutations in moderate-penetrance genes are more likely to be associated with an increased risk of breast cancer if encoding for the region in key functional domains of the proteins and are highly preserved within species [66]. An exception to the rule is the missense *ATM* c.7271T > G, a variant associated with a relative risk for breast cancer of more than 4 [67, 68], equivalent to that of a high-penetrance gene. Importantly, the risk of breast cancer appears increased twofold compared to truncating variants [69].

Cell cycle kinase 2 (CHEK2) participates in the DNA damage signal transduction. *CHEK2* is a moderately penetrant gene. The odds for breast cancer are 2.29 times higher for heterozygotes for the truncating variant compared to noncarriers [23]. For the missense *CHEK2* I157T mutation, the relative risk was less than 2—a risk more comparable to a low-penetrance gene [70]. Individual homozygotes for the c.1100delC *CHEK2* variant appear to have higher odds for breast cancer compared to heterozygotes (odds ratio 2.7 vs. 3.4, respectively) [71].

Recently, *BARD1*, *RAD51D*, and *MSH6* were identified as moderate-penetrance genes. The frequency of pathogenic mutation in each gene was less than 0.10% in the study by Couch et al. [23]. BRCA1 associated RING domain 1 (BARD1) and RAD51D are parts of homologous recombination DNA repair cell machinery. BARD1 stabilizes BRCA1, and it is essential for its expression [72]. *BARD1* mutations increase the odds for breast cancer by 2–3 times (CI 95% 1.29–3.73) [23]. RAD51D is one of the RAD51 recombinase paralogs and was thought to be a low-penetrance breast cancer gene [73]. The risk was found to be higher in the study by Couch et al. (odds ratio 3.07; CI 95% 1.17–9.44) [23]. *MSH6* is a gene encoding for a protein participating in mismatch DNA repair and is mainly associated with an increased risk for colorectal cancer (hereditary non-polyposis colorectal cancer) [74]. In the Couch et al. study, the risk for breast cancer was found to be moderately increased [23]. Finally, presence of significant family history of breast cancer can also modify risk in non-affected carriers of moderate-penetrance genes [65, 75, 76].

8.2.3   Clinical Utility

Detecting a germline mutation in a breast cancer predisposition gene may have implications in the management of an individual patient (therapeutics/tertiary prevention) or in the primary or secondary prevention counseling of an unaffected relative. The threshold for intervention is not well defined. The use of cumulative lifetime breast cancer risk suffers from inconsistencies in its definition/calculation (risk of ever developing cancer vs. remaining cancer risk based on individuals' age) [77]. Using a more short-term risk such as the 5-year breast cancer risk may be more appropriate in shared decision-making/counseling. An intervention appears rational when the 5-year breast cancer risk exceeds the risk in the general US population (1% in 5-years) or the highest population incidence in the general population (2% in 5-years for women 70–80 years old) [77]. The National Comprehensive Cancer Network (NCCN) [78] provides recommendations regarding primary prevention, and early detection of breast cancer in carriers of deleterious mutations is shown in Table 8.3.

8.2.3.1   High-Penetrance Genes

Primary Prevention
Several studies have established that RRM and RRSO significantly decrease the risk of breast and ovarian cancer in *BRCA1/2* carriers. More specifically, prospective (non-randomized) data from the Prevention and Observation of Surgical Endpoints (PROSE) consortium reveal a significant decrease in breast cancer incidence in *BRCA1/2* carriers with risk-reducing mastectomy (RRM) (0 vs. 7%) and risk-reducing salpingo-oophorectomy (RRSO) (no prior history of breast cancer: 11 vs. 21%, HR 0.54; there was no evidence of decreased risk in individuals with a prior diagnosis of breast cancer) [25]. There was a significant decrease in the

Table 8.3 Summary of National Comprehensive Cancer Network (NCCN) recommendations for deleterious gene mutations carriers; MRI = magnetic resonance imaging, N/A = not available, RRM = risk-reducing mastectomy, RRSO = risk-reducing salpingo-oophorectomy [78]

Gene	Breast cancer risk	Ovarian cancer risk	Other cancers	Recommendations for breast/ovarian cancer risk reduction
ATM[1]	Increased	Not increased	Unknown/insufficient evidence for prostate and pancreas cancer	• Annual mammogram/consider breast MRI starting at the age of 40 years • Consider RRM (based on family history)
BRCA1	Increased	Increased	Prostate	• Annual mammogram starting at the age of 30 years/annual breast MRI starting at the age of 25 years • Consider RRM • Recommend RRSO at the age of 35-40 years
BRCA2	Increased	Increased	Prostate, pancreas, melanoma	• Annual mammogram starting at the age of 30 years/annual breast MRI starting at the age of 25 years • Consider RRM • Recommend RRSO at the age of 35-40 years (can extend to 40-45 years)
BRIP1	Not increased	Increased	N/A	• Consider RRSO at the age of 45-50 years
CDH1	Increased	Not increased	Diffuse gastric cancer	• Annual mammogram/consider breast MRI starting at the age of 30 years • Consider RRM (based on family history)
CHEK2[2]	Increased	Not increased	Colon cancer	• Annual mammogram/consider breast MRI starting at the age of 40 years • Consider RRM (based on family history)
MSH6	Unknown/insufficient	Not increased	Colorectal cancer, endometrial cancer	• Breast cancer management based on family history
NBN[3]	Increased	Unknown/insufficient	Unknown/insufficient	• Annual mammogram/consider breast MRI starting at the age of 40 years

(continued)

Table 8.3 (continued)

Gene	Breast cancer risk	Ovarian cancer risk	Other cancers	Recommendations for breast/ovarian cancer risk reduction
NF1	Increased	Not increased	Gastrointestinal stromal tumors, malignant peripheral nerve sheath tumors	• Consider RRM (based on family history) • Annual mammogram starting at the age of 30 years/consider breast MRI starting at the age of 30–50 years
PALB2	Increased	Unknown/insufficient	Unknown/insufficient	• Consider RRM (based on family history) • Annual mammogram/consider breast MRI starting at the age of 30 years • Consider RRM (based on family history)
PTEN	Increased	Not increased	Thyroid cancer, endometrial cancer	• Annual mammogram/breast MRI starting at the age of 30–35 years • Consider RRM
RAD51C	Unknown	Increased	N/A	• Consider RRSO at the age of 45–50 years
RAD51D	Unknown	Increased	N/A	• Consider RRSO at the age of 45–50 years
STK11	Increased	Increased (non-epithelial)	Colorectal cancer	• Annual mammogram/breast MRI starting at the age of 25 years
P53	Increased	Not increased	Adrenocortical carcinoma, leukemia, brain tumors, soft tissue sarcomas	• Annual mammogram starting at the age of 30 years/annual breast MRI starting at the age of 20–29 years • Consider RRM

[1]The risk for missense variant c.7271T > G is higher compared to truncating mutations

[2]Risk is mainly increased for frameshift mutations

[3]Data exist mainly for the 657del5 Slavic truncating mutation

incidence of ovarian cancer with RRSO (72% for patients with no prior history of breast cancer and 85% for patients with a prior history of breast cancer). More importantly, RRSO led to a significantly improved overall survival (OS) in individuals with no and with prior breast cancer diagnosis (HR = 0.45 and 0.30 respectively), decreased breast cancer (HR = 0.44), and ovarian cancer-specific mortality (HR = 0.24) [25].

Prospective data on the role of prophylactic mastectomy in individuals with Cowden and Li-Fraumeni syndrome do not exist, but national guidelines recommend discussing this option with individuals screened positive for deleterious mutations [78].

Early Detection

Screening with mammography alone is considered to have an unacceptable rate of interval cancers in addition to high risk of detection of higher stage disease [79]. Using a screening protocol incorporating annual contrast-enhanced breast MRI, breast ultrasound and mammogram as well as semiannual clinical breast examination, Passaperuma et al. reported on an interval cancer rate was 2% (3% for BRCA1 carriers) [80]. No cancer was diagnosed in individuals younger than 30 years; the detection rate thereafter increased with increasing age. The sensitivity of the MRI is higher (86 vs. 19%) and increases with age. The specificity of mammogram was higher (97 vs. 90%). This strategy resulted in an annual breast cancer-specific mortality rate of 0.5%. In a non-randomized prospective study in *BRCA1/2* carriers of a screening strategy incorporating both breast MRI and mammography (comparison was a contemporary cohort of *BRCA1/2* carriers in North America not screened with breast MRI), the cumulative incidence of non-invasive and invasive breast cancer was comparable between MRI screened and unscreened individuals (5.1 vs. 1.6% $P = 0.63$ and 10.6 vs. 12.2% $P = 0.7$, respectively); stage migration was noted [27]. Screening with MRI decreased the risk of developing stage II–IV disease by 70%. Results from the prospective, non-randomized Dutch MRI screening study (MRISC) also confirm stage migration and improved metastasis-free survival but not overall survival [81]. There are to date no prospective data supporting an overall survival benefit with MRI screening for *BRCA1/2* mutation carriers; microsimulation models like MISCAN predict substantial decreases in mortality [82]. The American Cancer Society (ACS) recommends annual MRI testing as an adjunct to mammography in individuals with deleterious *BRCA1/2* mutations [83], and this recommendation is endorsed by both the NCCN and National Institute for Health and Care Excellence (NICE) guidelines.

High-quality prospective data regarding enhanced screening do not exist for syndromes associated with other high-penetrance genes, but national guidelines do recommend screening with mammography and MRI extrapolating from data in *BRCA1/2* mutations carriers. In a small observational study in 33 *p53* mutation carriers, the 3-year overall survival in the 18 individuals who elected enhanced screening was 100% versus 21% in the non-screened population ($P = 0.0155$), a finding that may be related to healthy user bias [84]. The potential benefit of screening protocols for Li-Fraumeni syndrome should be weighted against harms from increased sensitivity to diagnostic (and therapeutic) radiation and development of radiation-associated malignancies [85, 86].

Therapeutics

BRCA-positive breast cancers have an impaired homologous recombination DNA repair process and considered to be sensitive to DNA damage from cross-linking agents like platinum salts [87]. Phase II studies confirmed improved response rates with platinum agents in *BRCA* carriers, though progression-free survival (PFS) and OS appeared comparable between mutation carriers and noncarriers [88, 89]. Subgroup analysis of TNT, a randomized phase III study of carboplatin versus docetaxel in patients with advanced triple-negative breast cancer, points toward increased efficacy of carboplatin in *BRCA* mutation positive patients [90].

Homologous recombination DNA repair deficiency renders *BRCA*-deficient tumors dependent on alternative DNA repair pathways for survival (synthetic lethality), including base excision repair (BER). Poly (ADP-ribose) polymerase (PARP) is a key enzyme in the BER pathway [91]. PARP inhibitors can induce cell death in *BRCA*-deficient cancer cells [92, 93]. The PARP inhibitor olaparib as single-agent therapy has proven short-term activity in phase II studies in breast cancer patients harboring a deleterious *BRCA* mutation, with response rates ranging from 19 to 50% depending on the dose and the type of mutation [94, 95]. The Food and Drugs Administration (FDA) has approved olaparib for the treatment of metastatic, platinum-resistant ovarian cancer who has progressed after at least three prior systemic therapies in individuals harboring a deleterious germline mutation [96].

Preclinical studies reveal potential synergy between PARP inhibitors and platinum salts in *BRCA*-deficient breast cancer cells and/or animal models providing rationale for combination strategies [97, 98]. In a phase I/Ib trial, olaparib in combination with carboplatin in individuals with various tumors harboring a *BRCA* mutation was safe; the overall response rate was 50% [99]. Iniparib, another PARP inhibitor, in combination with gemcitabine and carboplatin improved short-term outcomes (response and clinical benefit rate) in patients with advanced, pretreated triple-negative breast cancer compared to chemotherapy alone [100], but the confirmatory trial was negative for a PFS and OS benefit [101]. These studies did not select patients based on the presence or not of a *BRCA* mutation, and a subgroup analysis based on the mutation status was not provided; further, iniparib was subsequently found to be a weak PARP inhibitor with decreased activity against homologous recombination deficient cells, potentially explaining negative results of the study [102].

As mentioned above, therapeutic radiotherapy may be omitted if not medically necessary in management of breast cancer in individuals with the Li-Fraumeni syndrome.

8.2.3.2 Moderate-Penetrance Genes

Clinical decision-making in cases of moderate-penetrance gene carriers is not straightforward. There is no high-quality clinical evidence guiding practitioners. Based on expert opinion, primary prevention or early detection should be discussed on an individual basis with pathogenic mutation carriers when individual short-term risk exceeds that of the average short-term risk in the general population [77]. As the lifetime risk of breast cancer in this population exceeds 20%, screening breast MRI should be included based on the ACS recommendations [83]. In the prospective Magnetic Resonance Imaging Breast Screening (MARIBS) study, 65% of the patients were included based on their family history of breast or ovarian cancer; the rest were either *BRCA* positive or were relatives of known carriers [103]. Even though in the complete cohort the sensitivity of breast MRI was superior to mammography, when *BRCA1* positive or relatives or known *BRCA1* carriers were excluded the sensitivity was the same in between the two screening methods.

Heterozygosity for *CHEK2* 1100delC has been associated with increased risk of breast cancer-specific death in patients with early invasive disease, but its usefulness for treatment decision-making (e.g., use of cytotoxic systemic therapy) is currently unclear [104].

8.3 Panel Testing Versus Sequential Single Gene Testing

Selecting a gene panel testing when considering a hereditary breast cancer syndrome has certain advantages. It is more cost-effective and time-efficient, but the VUS and gene variants with unclear clinical implications detection rate are higher. In a cohort of 278 patients with breast-ovarian cancer syndrome tested negative for a *BRCA* pathogenic mutation, 31 (11%) had a class 4 or 5 variant; of those, only 7 had a mutation in a high-penetrance gene [105]. In a large prospective cohort of *BRCA* mutation-negative individuals evaluated for hereditary breast-ovarian cancer, there was a change in management suggested for 52% of carriers of a non-*BRCA* pathogenic gene variant, mostly increased—breast or other—cancer surveillance [106]. Notably, 11 (17%) of the individuals carrying a mutation were found to have a hereditary colorectal cancer syndrome, most commonly Lynch syndrome. Single gene, from the other hand, carries the risk of testing fatigue and potentially loss of follow-up. Recently, updated NCCN guidelines included management suggestions for moderate-penetrance genes [78]. The decision for panel gene testing should be made when pre- or post-test consultation with a genetic counselor is available.

8.4 Conclusions

While identification of individuals carrying a pathogenic high-penetrance gene mutation like *BRCA* has profound implications in clinical management, the potential of discovering either VUS or moderate/low-penetrance alterations through widespread adoption of panel gene testing can lead to overestimation of individual risk and interventions with no proven benefit. Genetic testing should be continued to offer to patients at high risk [78] in order to make optimal decisions for patients and their families.

References

1. Collaborative Group on Hormonal Factors in Breast C. (2001) Familial breast cancer: collaborative reanalysis of individual data from 52 epidemiological studies including 58,209 women with breast cancer and 101,986 women without the disease. Lancet 358(9291): 1389–1399. doi:10.1016/S0140-6736(01)06524-2
2. Lindor NM, McMaster ML, Lindor CJ, Greene MH (2008) Concise handbook of familial cancer susceptibility syndromes, 2nd edn. JNCI Monogr (38):3–93. doi:10.1093/jncimonographs/lgn001
3. Petrucelli N, Daly MB, Feldman GL (2010) Hereditary breast and ovarian cancer due to mutations in BRCA1 and BRCA2. Genet Med 12(5):245–259
4. Ford D, Easton DF, Stratton M, Narod S, Goldgar D, Devilee P et al (1998) Genetic heterogeneity and penetrance analysis of the BRCA1 and BRCA2 genes in breast cancer families. Am J Hum Genet 62(3):676–689. http://dx.doi.org/10.1086/301749
5. Whittemore AS, Gong G, Itnyre J (1997) Prevalence and contribution of BRCA1 mutations in breast cancer and ovarian cancer: results from three U.S. population-based case-control studies of ovarian cancer. Am J Hum Genet 60(3):496–504
6. Claus EB, Schildkraut JM, Thompson WD, Risch NJ (1996) The genetic attributable risk of breast and ovarian cancer. Cancer 77(11):2318–2324. doi:10.1002/(SICI)1097-0142 (19960601)77:11<2318:AID-CNCR21>3.0.CO;2-Z
7. John EM, Miron A, Gong G, Phipps AI, Felberg A, Li FP et al (2007) Prevalence of pathogenic BRCA1 mutation carriers in 5 US racial/ethnic groups. JAMA 298(24): 2869–2876. doi:10.1001/jama.298.24.2869
8. Szabo CI, King MC (1997) Population genetics of BRCA1 and BRCA2. Am J Hum Genet 60(5):1013–1020
9. Roa BB, Boyd AA, Volcik K, Richards CS (1996) Ashkenazi Jewish population frequencies for common mutations in BRCA1 and BRCA2. Nat Genet 14(2):185–187
10. Moslehi R, Chu W, Karlan B, Fishman D, Risch H, Fields A et al (2000) *BRCA1* and *BRCA2* Mutation Analysis of 208 Ashkenazi Jewish Women with Ovarian Cancer. Am J Hum Genet 66(4):1259–1272. doi:10.1086/302853
11. King M-C, Marks JH, Mandell JB (2003) Breast and ovarian cancer risks due to inherited mutations in BRCA1 and BRCA2. Science 302(5645):643–646. doi:10.1126/science. 1088759
12. Chen S, Parmigiani G (2007) Meta-analysis of BRCA1 and BRCA2 penetrance. J Clin Oncol 25(11):1329–1333. doi:10.1200/jco.2006.09.1066
13. Evans DG, Shenton A, Woodward E, Lalloo F, Howell A, Maher ER (2008) Penetrance estimates for BRCA1 and BRCA2 based on genetic testing in a Clinical Cancer Genetics service setting: risks of breast/ovarian cancer quoted should reflect the cancer burden in the family. BMC Cancer 8:155. doi:10.1186/1471-2407-8-155

14. Antoniou A, Pharoah PD, Narod S, Risch HA, Eyfjord JE, Hopper JL et al (2003) Average risks of breast and ovarian cancer associated with BRCA1 or BRCA2 mutations detected in case series unselected for family history: a combined analysis of 22 studies. Am J Hum Genet 72(5):1117–1130. doi:10.1086/375033

15. Mavaddat N, Peock S, Frost D, Ellis S, Platte R, Fineberg E et al (2013) Cancer risks for BRCA1 and BRCA2 mutation carriers: results from prospective analysis of EMBRACE. J Natl Cancer Inst 105(11):812–822. doi:10.1093/jnci/djt095

16. Mavaddat N, Barrowdale D, Andrulis IL, Domchek SM, Eccles D, Nevanlinna H et al (2012) Pathology of breast and ovarian cancers among BRCA1 and BRCA2 mutation carriers: results from the Consortium of Investigators of Modifiers of BRCA1/2 (CIMBA). Cancer Epidemiol Biomark Prev 21(1):134–147. doi:10.1158/1055-9965.EPI-11-0775

17. Malkin D (1994) Germline p53 mutations and heritable cancer. Annu Rev Genet 28(1): 443–465. doi:10.1146/annurev.ge.28.120194.002303

18. Nelen MR, Padberg GW, Peeters EAJ, Lin AY, Bvd Helm, Frants RR et al (1996) Localization of the gene for Cowden disease to chromosome 10q22-23. Nat Genet 13(1): 114–116

19. Hemminki A, Markie D, Tomlinson I, Avizienyte E, Roth S, Loukola A et al (1998) A serine/threonine kinase gene defective in Peutz-Jeghers syndrome. Nature 391(6663): 184–187. doi:10.1038/34432

20. Lustbader ED, Williams WR, Bondy ML, Strom S, Strong LC (1992) Segregation analysis of cancer in families of childhood soft-tissue-sarcoma patients. Am J Hum Genet 51(2): 344–356

21. Pharoah PD, Guilford P, Caldas C, International Gastric Cancer Linkage C (2001) Incidence of gastric cancer and breast cancer in CDH1 (E-cadherin) mutation carriers from hereditary diffuse gastric cancer families. Gastroenterology 121(6):1348–1353

22. Stadler ZK, Thom P, Robson ME, Weitzel JN, Kauff ND, Hurley KE et al (2010) Genome-Wide Association Studies of Cancer. J Clin Oncol 28(27):4255–4267. doi:10.1200/JCO.2009.25.7816

23. Couch FJ, Hu C, Lilyquist J, Shimelis H, Akinhanmi M, Na J, Polley EC, Hart SN, McFarland R, LaDuca H, Huether R, Goldgar DE, Dolinsky JS (eds) (2016) Breast cancer risks associated with mutations in cancer predisposition genes identified by clinical genetic testing of 60,000 breast cancer patients. In: 39th San Antonio breast cancer symposium, San Antonio, TX, USA

24. Thompson D, Easton D (2004) The genetic epidemiology of breast cancer genes. J Mammary Gland Biol Neoplasia 9(3):221–236. doi:10.1023/B:JOMG.0000048770.90334.3b

25. Domchek SM, Friebel TM, Singer CF, Evans DG, Lynch HT, Isaacs C et al (2010) Association of risk-reducing surgery in BRCA1 or BRCA2 mutation carriers with cancer risk and mortality. JAMA, J Am Med Assoc 304(9):967–975. doi:10.1001/jama.2010.1237

26. Kriege M, Brekelmans CT, Boetes C, Besnard PE, Zonderland HM, Obdeijn IM et al (2004) Efficacy of MRI and mammography for breast-cancer screening in women with a familial or genetic predisposition. N Engl J Med 351(5):427–437. doi:10.1056/NEJMoa031759

27. Warner E, Hill K, Causer P, Plewes D, Jong R, Yaffe M et al (2011) Prospective study of breast cancer incidence in women with a BRCA1 or BRCA2 mutation under surveillance with and without magnetic resonance imaging. J Clin Oncol 29(13):1664–1669. doi:10.1200/JCO.2009.27.0835

28. Association for Molecular Pathology v. Myriad Genetics, Inc. 569 U.S. (2013) United States Supreme Court. https://supreme.justia.com/cases/federal/us/569/12-398. Accessed 2 Sept 2016

29. Haddow J, Palomaki GE (2003) ACCE: a model process for evaluating data on emerging genetic tests. In: Khoury MJLJ, Burke W (eds) Human genome epidemiology: a scientific foundation for using genetic information to improve health and prevent disease. Oxford University Press, Oxford, UK, pp 217–233

30. Lincoln SE, Kobayashi Y, Anderson MJ, Yang S, Desmond AJ, Mills MA et al (2015) A systematic comparison of traditional and multigene panel testing for hereditary breast and

ovarian cancer genes in more than 1000 patients. J Mol Diagn 17(5):533–544. doi:10.1016/j.
jmoldx.2015.04.009

31. Couch FJ, Nathanson KL, Offit K (2014) Two decades after BRCA: setting paradigms in
    personalized cancer care and prevention. Science 343(6178):1466–1470. doi:10.1126/
    science.1251827

32. Easton DF, Pharoah PD, Antoniou AC, Tischkowitz M, Tavtigian SV, Nathanson KL et al
    (2015) Gene-panel sequencing and the prediction of breast-cancer risk. N Engl J Med 372
    (23):2243–2257. doi:10.1056/NEJMsr1501341

33. Plon SE, Eccles DM, Easton D, Foulkes WD, Genuardi M, Greenblatt MS et al (2008)
    Sequence variant classification and reporting: recommendations for improving the interpre-
    tation of cancer susceptibility genetic test results. Hum Mutat 29(11):1282–1291. doi:10.
    1002/humu.20880

34. Walker LC, Whiley PJ, Couch FJ, Farrugia DJ, Healey S, Eccles DM et al (2010) Detection
    of splicing aberrations caused by BRCA1 and BRCA2 sequence variants encoding missense
    substitutions: implications for prediction of pathogenicity. Hum Mutat 31(6):E1484–E1505.
    doi:10.1002/humu.21267

35. Thompson BA, Spurdle AB, Plazzer JP, Greenblatt MS, Akagi K, Al-Mulla F et al (2014)
    Application of a 5-tiered scheme for standardized classification of 2,360 unique mismatch
    repair gene variants in the InSiGHT locus-specific database. Nat Genet 46(2):107–115.
    doi:10.1038/ng.2854

36. Richards CS, Bale S, Bellissimo DB, Das S, Grody WW, Hegde MR et al (2008) ACMG
    recommendations for standards for interpretation and reporting of sequence variations:
    revisions 2007. Genet Med 10(4):294–300. doi:10.1097/GIM.0b013e31816b5cae

37. Easton DF, Deffenbaugh AM, Pruss D, Frye C, Wenstrup RJ, Allen-Brady K et al (2007) A
    systematic genetic assessment of 1,433 sequence variants of unknown clinical significance in
    the BRCA1 and BRCA2 breast cancer-predisposition genes. Am J Hum Genet 81(5):873–
    883. doi:10.1086/521032

38. Goldgar DE, Easton DF, Deffenbaugh AM, Monteiro AN, Tavtigian SV, Couch FJ et al
    (2004) Integrated evaluation of DNA sequence variants of unknown clinical significance:
    application to BRCA1 and BRCA2. Am J Hum Genet 75(4):535–544. doi:10.1086/424388

39. Tavtigian SV, Greenblatt MS, Lesueur F, Byrnes GB, Group IUGVW (2008) In silico
    analysis of missense substitutions using sequence-alignment based methods. Hum Mutat
    29(11):1327–1336. doi:10.1002/humu.20892

40. Vallee MP, Francy TC, Judkins MK, Babikyan D, Lesueur F, Gammon A et al (2012)
    Classification of missense substitutions in the BRCA genes: a database dedicated to Ex-UVs.
    Hum Mutat 33(1):22–28. doi:10.1002/humu.21629

41. Thompson D, Easton DF, Goldgar DE (2003) A full-likelihood method for the evaluation of
    causality of sequence variants from family data. Am J Hum Genet 73(3):652–655. doi:10.
    1086/378100

42. Chenevix-Trench G, Healey S, Lakhani S, Waring P, Cummings M, Brinkworth R et al
    (2006) Genetic and histopathologic evaluation of BRCA1 and BRCA2 DNA sequence
    variants of unknown clinical significance. Cancer Res 66(4):2019–2027. doi:10.1158/0008-
    5472.CAN-05-3546

43. Spurdle AB, Lakhani SR, Healey S, Parry S, Da Silva LM, Brinkworth R et al (2008)
    Clinical classification of BRCA1 and BRCA2 DNA sequence variants: the value of
    cytokeratin profiles and evolutionary analysis—a report from the kConFab Investigators.
    J Clin Oncol 26(10):1657–1663. doi:10.1200/JCO.2007.13.2779

44. Yeo G, Burge CB (2004) Maximum entropy modeling of short sequence motifs with
    applications to RNA splicing signals. J Comput Biol 11(2–3):377–394. doi:10.1089/
    1066527041410418

45. Guidugli L, Pankratz VS, Singh N, Thompson J, Erding CA, Engel C et al (2013) A
    classification model for BRCA2 DNA binding domain missense variants based on

homology-directed repair activity. Cancer Res 73(1):265–275. doi:10.1158/0008-5472. CAN-12-2081

46. Lindor NM, Guidugli L, Wang X, Vallee MP, Monteiro AN, Tavtigian S et al (2012) A review of a multifactorial probability-based model for classification of BRCA1 and BRCA2 variants of uncertain significance (VUS). Hum Mutat 33(1):8–21. doi:10.1002/humu.21627

47. Rebbeck TR, Mitra N, Wan F, Sinilnikova OM, Healey S, McGuffog L et al (2015) Association of type and location of BRCA1 and BRCA2 mutations with risk of breast and ovarian cancer. JAMA 313(13):1347–1361. doi:10.1001/jama.2014.5985

48. Spurdle AB, Whiley PJ, Thompson B, Feng B, Healey S, Brown MA et al (2012) BRCA1 R1699Q variant displaying ambiguous functional abrogation confers intermediate breast and ovarian cancer risk. J Med Genet 49(8):525–532. doi:10.1136/jmedgenet-2012-101037

49. Thompson D, Easton D, Breast Cancer Linkage C. (2001) Variation in cancer risks, by mutation position, in BRCA2 mutation carriers. Am J Hum Genet 68(2):410–419. doi:10. 1086/318181

50. Michailidou K, Hall P, Gonzalez-Neira A, Ghoussaini M, Dennis J, Milne RL et al (2013) Large-scale genotyping identifies 41 new loci associated with breast cancer risk. Nat Genet 45(4):353–361, 61e1-2. doi:10.1038/ng.2563

51. Antoniou AC, Beesley J, McGuffog L, Sinilnikova OM, Healey S, Neuhausen SL et al (2010) Common breast cancer susceptibility alleles and the risk of breast cancer for BRCA1 and BRCA2 mutation carriers: implications for risk prediction. Cancer Res 70(23): 9742–9754. doi:10.1158/0008-5472.CAN-10-1907

52. Antoniou AC, Spurdle AB, Sinilnikova OM, Healey S, Pooley KA, Schmutzler RK et al (2008) Common breast cancer-predisposition alleles are associated with breast cancer risk in BRCA1 and BRCA2 mutation carriers. Am J Hum Genet 82(4):937–948. doi:10.1016/j. ajhg.2008.02.008

53. Rowan E, Poll A, Narod SA (2007) A prospective study of breast cancer risk in relatives of BRCA1/BRCA2 mutation carriers. J Med Genet 44(8):e89; author reply e8

54. Domchek SM, Gaudet MM, Stopfer JE, Fleischaut MH, Powers J, Kauff N et al (2010) Breast cancer risks in individuals testing negative for a known family mutation in BRCA1 or BRCA2. Breast Cancer Res Treat 119(2):409–414. doi:10.1007/s10549-009-0611-y

55. Korde LA, Mueller CM, Loud JT, Struewing JP, Nichols K, Greene MH et al (2011) No evidence of excess breast cancer risk among mutation-negative women from BRCA mutation-positive families. Breast Cancer Res Treat 125(1):169–173. doi:10.1007/s10549-010-0923-y

56. Harvey SL, Milne RL, McLachlan SA, Friedlander ML, Birch KE, Weideman P et al (2011) Prospective study of breast cancer risk for mutation negative women from BRCA1 or BRCA2 mutation positive families. Breast Cancer Res Treat 130(3):1057–1061. doi:10. 1007/s10549-011-1733-6

57. Malkin D, Li FP, Strong LC, Fraumeni JF Jr, Nelson CE, Kim DH et al (1990) Germ line p53 mutations in a familial syndrome of breast cancer, sarcomas, and other neoplasms. Science 250(4985):1233–1238

58. Hwang SJ, Lozano G, Amos CI, Strong LC (2003) Germline p53 mutations in a cohort with childhood sarcoma: sex differences in cancer risk. Am J Hum Genet 72(4):975–983. doi:10. 1086/374567

59. Tan MH, Mester JL, Ngeow J, Rybicki LA, Orloff MS, Eng C (2012) Lifetime cancer risks in individuals with germline PTEN mutations. Clin Cancer Res 18(2):400–407. doi:10.1158/ 1078-0432.CCR-11-2283

60. Hearle N, Schumacher V, Menko FH, Olschwang S, Boardman LA, Gille JJ et al (2006) Frequency and spectrum of cancers in the Peutz-Jeghers syndrome. Clin Cancer Res 12(10): 3209–3215. doi:10.1158/1078-0432.CCR-06-0083

61. Casadei S, Norquist BM, Walsh T, Stray S, Mandell JB, Lee MK et al (2011) Contribution of inherited mutations in the BRCA2-interacting protein PALB2 to familial breast cancer. Cancer Res 71(6):2222–2229. doi:10.1158/0008-5472.CAN-10-3958

62. Rahman N, Seal S, Thompson D, Kelly P, Renwick A, Elliott A et al (2007) PALB2, which encodes a BRCA2-interacting protein, is a breast cancer susceptibility gene. Nat Genet 39 (2):165–167. URL:http://www.nature.com/ng/journal/v39/n2/suppinfo/ng1959_S1.html

63. Erkko H, Dowty JG, Nikkila J, Syrjakoski K, Mannermaa A, Pylkas K et al (2008) Penetrance analysis of the PALB2 c.1592delT founder mutation. Clin Cancer Res 14(14): 4667–4671. doi:10.1158/1078-0432.CCR-08-0210

64. Southey MC, Teo ZL, Dowty JG, Odefrey FA, Park DJ, Tischkowitz M et al (2010) A PALB2 mutation associated with high risk of breast cancer. Breast Cancer Res 12(6):R109. doi:10.1186/bcr2796

65. Antoniou AC, Casadei S, Heikkinen T, Barrowdale D, Pylkas K, Roberts J et al (2014) Breast-cancer risk in families with mutations in PALB2. N Engl J Med 371(6):497–506. doi:10.1056/NEJMoa1400382

66. Le Calvez-Kelm F, Lesueur F, Damiola F, Vallee M, Voegele C, Babikyan D et al (2011) Rare, evolutionarily unlikely missense substitutions in CHEK2 contribute to breast cancer susceptibility: results from a breast cancer family registry case-control mutation-screening study. Breast Cancer Res 13(1):R6. doi:10.1186/bcr2810

67. Mitui M, Nahas SA, Du LT, Yang Z, Lai CH, Nakamura K et al (2009) Functional and computational assessment of missense variants in the ataxia-telangiectasia mutated (ATM) gene: mutations with increased cancer risk. Hum Mutat 30(1):12–21. doi:10.1002/humu.20805

68. Bernstein JL, Teraoka S, Southey MC, Jenkins MA, Andrulis IL, Knight JA et al (2006) Population-based estimates of breast cancer risks associated with ATM gene variants c.7271T > G and c.1066-6T > G (IVS10-6T > G) from the Breast Cancer Family Registry. Hum Mutat 27(11):1122–1128. doi:10.1002/humu.20415

69. Goldgar DE, Healey S, Dowty JG, Da Silva L, Chen X, Spurdle AB et al (2011) Rare variants in the ATM gene and risk of breast cancer. Breast Cancer Res 13(4):R73. doi:10.1186/bcr2919

70. Kilpivaara O, Vahteristo P, Falck J, Syrjakoski K, Eerola H, Easton D et al (2004) CHEK2 variant I157T may be associated with increased breast cancer risk. Int J Cancer 111(4): 543–547. doi:10.1002/ijc.20299

71. Huijts PE, Hollestelle A, Balliu B, Houwing-Duistermaat JJ, Meijers CM, Blom JC et al (2014) CHEK2*1100delC homozygosity in the Netherlands–prevalence and risk of breast and lung cancer. Eur J Hum Genet 22(1):46–51. doi:10.1038/ejhg.2013.85

72. Wu LC, Wang ZW, Tsan JT, Spillman MA, Phung A, Xu XL et al (1996) Identification of a RING protein that can interact in vivo with the BRCA1 gene product. Nat Genet 14(4): 430–440. doi:10.1038/ng1296-430

73. Loveday C, Turnbull C, Ramsay E, Hughes D, Ruark E, Frankum JR et al (2011) Germline mutations in RAD51D confer susceptibility to ovarian cancer. Nat Genet 43(9):879–882. doi:10.1038/ng.893

74. Baglietto L, Lindor NM, Dowty JG, White DM, Wagner A, Gomez Garcia EB et al (2010) Risks of Lynch syndrome cancers for MSH6 mutation carriers. J Natl Cancer Inst 102 (3):193–201. doi:10.1093/jnci/djp473

75. Adank MA, Verhoef S, Oldenburg RA, Schmidt MK, Hooning MJ, Martens JW et al (2013) Excess breast cancer risk in first degree relatives of CHEK2 *1100delC positive familial breast cancer cases. Eur J Cancer 49(8):1993–1999. doi:10.1016/j.ejca.2013.01.009

76. Consortium CBCC-C (2004) CHEK2*1100delC and susceptibility to breast cancer: a collaborative analysis involving 10,860 breast cancer cases and 9,065 controls from 10 studies. Am J Hum Genet 74(6):1175–1182. doi:10.1086/421251

77. Tung N, Domchek SM, Stadler Z, Nathanson KL, Couch F, Garber JE et al (2016) Counselling framework for moderate-penetrance cancer-susceptibility mutations. Nat Rev Clin Oncol 13(9):581–588. doi:10.1038/nrclinonc.2016.90

78. Genetic/Familial High-Risk Assessment: Breast and Ovarian v2.2017. National Comprehensive Cancer Network (2016) https://www.nccn.org/professionals/physician_gls/pdf/genetics_screening.pdf. Accessed 9 Jan 2017

79. Warner E, Messersmith H, Causer P, Eisen A, Shumak R, Plewes D (2008) Systematic review: using magnetic resonance imaging to screen women at high risk for breast cancer. Ann Intern Med 148(9):671–679

80. Passaperuma K, Warner E, Causer PA, Hill KA, Messner S, Wong JW et al (2012) Long-term results of screening with magnetic resonance imaging in women with BRCA mutations. Br J Cancer 107(1):24–30. doi:10.1038/bjc.2012.204

81. Saadatmand S, Obdeijn IM, Rutgers EJ, Oosterwijk JC, Tollenaar RA, Woldringh GH et al (2015) Survival benefit in women with BRCA1 mutation or familial risk in the MRI screening study (MRISC). Int J Cancer 137(7):1729–1738. doi:10.1002/ijc.29534

82. Heijnsdijk EA, Warner E, Gilbert FJ, Tilanus-Linthorst MM, Evans G, Causer PA et al (2012) Differences in natural history between breast cancers in BRCA1 and BRCA2 mutation carriers and effects of MRI screening-MRISC, MARIBS, and Canadian studies combined. Cancer Epidemiol Biomark Prev 21(9):1458–1468. doi:10.1158/1055-9965.EPI-11-1196

83. Saslow D, Boetes C, Burke W, Harms S, Leach MO, Lehman CD et al (2007) American Cancer Society guidelines for breast screening with MRI as an adjunct to mammography. CA Cancer J Clin 57(2):75–89

84. Villani A, Tabori U, Schiffman J, Shlien A, Beyene J, Druker H et al (2011) Biochemical and imaging surveillance in germline TP53 mutation carriers with Li-Fraumeni syndrome: a prospective observational study. Lancet Oncol 12(6):559–567. doi:10.1016/S1470-2045(11)70119-X

85. Evans DG, Birch JM, Ramsden RT, Sharif S, Baser ME (2006) Malignant transformation and new primary tumours after therapeutic radiation for benign disease: substantial risks in certain tumour prone syndromes. J Med Genet 43(4):289–294. doi:10.1136/jmg.2005.036319

86. Varley JM (2003) Germline TP53 mutations and Li-Fraumeni syndrome. Hum Mutat 21(3):313–320. doi:10.1002/humu.10185

87. Kennedy RD, Quinn JE, Mullan PB, Johnston PG, Harkin DP (2004) The role of BRCA1 in the cellular response to chemotherapy. J Natl Cancer Inst 96(22):1659–1668. doi:10.1093/jnci/djh312

88. Isakoff SJ, Mayer EL, He L, Traina TA, Carey LA, Krag KJ et al (2015) TBCRC009: a multicenter phase ii clinical trial of platinum monotherapy with biomarker assessment in metastatic triple-negative breast cancer. J Clin Oncol 33(17):1902–1909. doi:10.1200/JCO.2014.57.6660

89. Byrski T, Dent R, Blecharz P, Foszczynska-Kloda M, Gronwald J, Huzarski T et al (2012) Results of a phase II open-label, non-randomized trial of cisplatin chemotherapy in patients with BRCA1-positive metastatic breast cancer. Breast Cancer Res 14(4):R110. doi:10.1186/bcr3231

90. Tutt A, Ellis P, Kilburn L, Gilett C, Pinder S, Abraham J et al (2015) The TNT trial: A randomized phase III trial of carboplatin (C) compared with docetaxel (D) for patients with metastatic or recurrent locally advanced triple negative or BRCA1/2 breast cancer (CRUK/07/012). Cancer Res 75:2. doi:10.1158/1538-7445.sabcs14-s3-01

91. Morales J, Li L, Fattah FJ, Dong Y, Bey EA, Patel M et al (2014) Review of poly (ADP-ribose) polymerase (PARP) mechanisms of action and rationale for targeting in cancer and other diseases. Crit Rev Eukaryot Gene Expr 24(1):15–28

92. Bryant HE, Schultz N, Thomas HD, Parker KM, Flower D, Lopez E et al (2005) Specific killing of BRCA2-deficient tumours with inhibitors of poly(ADP-ribose) polymerase. Nature 434(7035):913–917. doi:10.1038/nature03443

93. Farmer H, McCabe N, Lord CJ, Tutt AN, Johnson DA, Richardson TB et al (2005) Targeting the DNA repair defect in BRCA mutant cells as a therapeutic strategy. Nature 434 (7035):917–921. doi:10.1038/nature03445

94. Tutt A, Robson M, Garber JE, Domchek SM, Audeh MW, Weitzel JN et al (2010) Oral poly (ADP-ribose) polymerase inhibitor olaparib in patients with BRCA1 or BRCA2 mutations and advanced breast cancer: a proof-of-concept trial. Lancet 376(9737):235–244. doi:10. 1016/S0140-6736(10)60892-6

95. Fong PC, Boss DS, Yap TA, Tutt A, Wu P, Mergui-Roelvink M et al (2009) Inhibition of poly(ADP-ribose) polymerase in tumors from BRCA mutation carriers. N Engl J Med 361 (2):123–134. doi:10.1056/NEJMoa0900212

96. Olaparib. United States Food and Drug Administration (FDA) (2014) http://www.fda.gov/Drugs/InformationOnDrugs/ApprovedDrugs/ucm427598.htm. Accessed 11 Nov 2016

97. Evers B, Drost R, Schut E, de Bruin M, van der Burg E, Derksen PW et al (2008) Selective inhibition of BRCA2-deficient mammary tumor cell growth by AZD2281 and cisplatin. Clin Cancer Res 14(12):3916–3925. doi:10.1158/1078-0432.CCR-07-4953

98. Rottenberg S, Jaspers JE, Kersbergen A, van der Burg E, Nygren AO, Zander SA et al (2008) High sensitivity of BRCA1-deficient mammary tumors to the PARP inhibitor AZD2281 alone and in combination with platinum drugs. Proc Natl Acad Sci U S A. 105 (44):17079–17084. doi:10.1073/pnas.0806092105

99. Lee JM, Hays JL, Annunziata CM, Noonan AM, Minasian L, Zujewski JA et al (2014) Phase I/Ib study of olaparib and carboplatin in BRCA1 or BRCA2 mutation-associated breast or ovarian cancer with biomarker analyses. J Natl Cancer Inst 106(6):dju089. doi:10. 1093/jnci/dju089

100. O'Shaughnessy J, Osborne C, Pippen JE, Yoffe M, Patt D, Rocha C et al (2011) Iniparib plus chemotherapy in metastatic triple-negative breast cancer. N Engl J Med 364(3):205–214. doi:10.1056/NEJMoa1011418

101. O'Shaughnessy J, Schwartzberg L, Danso MA, Miller KD, Rugo HS, Neubauer M et al (2014) Phase III study of iniparib plus gemcitabine and carboplatin versus gemcitabine and carboplatin in patients with metastatic triple-negative breast cancer. J Clin Oncol 32 (34):3840–3847. doi:10.1200/JCO.2014.55.2984

102. Wang YQ, Wang PY, Wang YT, Yang GF, Zhang A, Miao ZH (2016) An update on poly (ADP-ribose)polymerase-1 (PARP-1) inhibitors: opportunities and challenges in cancer therapy. J Med Chem. doi:10.1021/acs.jmedchem.6b00055

103. Leach MO, Boggis CR, Dixon AK, Easton DF, Eeles RA, Evans DG et al (2005) Screening with magnetic resonance imaging and mammography of a UK population at high familial risk of breast cancer: a prospective multicentre cohort study (MARIBS). Lancet 365 (9473):1769–1778. doi:10.1016/S0140-6736(05)66481-1

104. Weischer M, Nordestgaard BG, Pharoah P, Bolla MK, Nevanlinna H, Van't Veer LJ et al (2012) CHEK2*1100delC heterozygosity in women with breast cancer associated with early death, breast cancer-specific death, and increased risk of a second breast cancer. J Clin Oncol 30(35):4308–4316. doi:10.1200/JCO.2012.42.7336

105. Maxwell KN, Wubbenhorst B, D'Andrea K, Garman B, Long JM, Powers J et al (2015) Prevalence of mutations in a panel of breast cancer susceptibility genes in BRCA1/2-negative patients with early-onset breast cancer. Genet Med. 17(8):630–638. doi:10.1038/gim.2014.176

106. Desmond A, Kurian AW, Gabree M, Mills MA, Anderson MJ, Kobayashi Y et al (2015) Clinical actionability of multigene panel testing for hereditary breast and ovarian cancer risk assessment. JAMA Oncol. 1(7):943–951. doi:10.1001/jamaoncol.2015.2690

Advances in Endocrine Therapy for Postmenopausal Metastatic Breast Cancer

9

Lisa E. Flaum and William J. Gradishar

Contents

L. E. Flaum · W. J. Gradishar (✉)
Robert H. Lurie Comprehensive Cancer Center of Northwestern University,
Chicago, IL, USA
e-mail: wgradish@nm.org

© Springer International Publishing AG 2018
W. J. Gradishar (ed.), *Optimizing Breast Cancer Management*, Cancer Treatment
and Research 173, https://doi.org/10.1007/978-3-319-70197-4_9

Abstract

A majority of breast cancers are hormone receptor (HR) positive and are responsive to various types of hormone manipulation. Endocrine therapy is the preferred first-line therapy for patients with advanced estrogen receptor (ER) positive, HER2-negative breast cancer who do not have symptomatic visceral disease. Endocrine therapy is often continued in the second- and third-line setting, with chemotherapy deferred until tumor becomes endocrine therapy refractory and/or a visceral crisis in imminent. Therapeutic options vary based on clinical presentation and include single-agent therapies such as tamoxifen, aromatase inhibitors and fulvestrant, and combination therapies options. Over the past few years, multiple trials have shown significant improvement in outcomes when endocrine therapy is combined with CDK 4/6 inhibitors or mTOR inhibitors. Improved efficacy comes at a cost of a modest increase in toxicity. Mechanisms of ER resistance have been defined leading to multiple strategies to improve efficacy and overcome resistance. These include the combination therapies options mentioned above and other novel drugs that are in development. This review will summarize the existing literature regarding endocrine therapy in postmenopausal metastatic breast cancer and outline treatment approaches in the first-line metastatic setting and beyond.

Keywords

Endocrine therapy · Advanced breast cancer · CK 4/6 inhibitors
mTOR inhibitors

9.1 Background

Hormonal manipulation has been an established paradigm in the treatment of breast cancer for over 100 years. Early trials demonstrated the regression of advanced breast cancer after oophorectomy or ovarian radiation [1]. It has since been elucidated that approximately 70% of breast cancers are hormone receptor (HR) positive. Although a majority of breast cancers are curable, $\sim$20–30% of patients present with denovo metastatic disease or progress to metastatic disease follow an early stage diagnosis. Treatment of metastatic disease is influenced by menopausal status, HR status, as well as other molecular features. This discussion will focus on the postmenopausal patient with HR-positive, metastatic breast cancer (MBC).

Endocrine therapy is the preferred choice as first-line therapy for patients with advanced estrogen receptor (ER) positive, HER2-negative breast cancer who do not have symptomatic visceral disease. Endocrine therapies work through various mechanisms including decreasing estrogen production (aromatase inhibitors), blocking signaling through the estrogen receptor (tamoxifen), or antagonizing the receptor itself (fulvestrant). First-line endocrine therapy is continued until disease progression or unacceptable toxicity. A change to second-line endocrine therapy can be considered at time of disease progression. Chemotherapy is typically recommended when the benefit of endocrine therapy lessens (with each prior endocrine therapy), the tumor becomes endocrine therapy refractory, and/or a visceral crisis is imminent. Although metastatic ER-positive breast cancers can respond well to sequential endocrine therapies, most patients will become resistant to these therapies, eventually require chemotherapy, and inevitably die of their disease. Mechanisms of ER resistance have been defined, leading to the development of novel therapies to improve efficacy and overcome resistance, including CDK 4/6 inhibitors, mTOR inhibitors, and others.

9.2   Evolution of Endocrine Therapy for Advanced Breast Cancer

The selective estrogen receptor modulator (SERM), tamoxifen, was approved in the 1970s as an effective therapy for patients with ER-positive MBC [2, 3]. Tamoxifen was shown to be superior to older drugs such as high-dose, oral medroxyprogesterone acetate as initial therapy for patients with metastatic breast cancers, with clinical response in up to one-third of patients [4]. Concerning side effects of tamoxifen, including thromboembolic disease and endometrial cancer, are related to the partial agonist features of the drug. Aromatase inhibitors (AIs) subsequently emerged as an alternative to tamoxifen in the first- and second-line setting for patients with ER-positive, MBC. AIs block the enzyme aromatase that prevents peripheral conversion of androgens to estrogen. AIs lack the agonistic properties of tamoxifen and minimize the risk of thromboembolic disease and endometrial malignancies. AIs were shown to be superior to megestrol acetate as second-line therapy of advanced ER-positive breast cancer following tamoxifen and superior to tamoxifen in the first-line setting [5–11]. A 2006 meta-analysis of 23-randomized trials with anastrozole, letrozole, or exemestane demonstrated improvement in overall survival (OS) compared to tamoxifen [12]. Subsequent studies compared AIs in the first- and second-line setting, and there is no data to suggest that one AI is superior to others [13, 14]. Based on this data, AI therapy has become a standard of care for first- and second-line therapy of postmenopausal patients with ER-positive, MBC.

Fulvestrant is another effective option in this patient population. Fulvestrant is an estrogen receptor antagonist that blocks ER dimerization, increases ER turnover, and accelerates degradation of the receptor [15]. Fulvestrant, initially studied at a dose of 250 mg, was compared to tamoxifen in the first-line, advanced disease setting and shown to have similar efficacy in ER-positive patients [16]. The 250 mg dose of fulvestrant was also found to have a similar clinical benefit rate compared to anastrozole in the second-line treatment of postmenopausal women with MBC [17, 18] and similar efficacy compared to exemestane in women treated with prior AI therapy [19]. OS was similar, 27.4 and 27.7 months for fulvestrant and anastrozole, respectively [20]. A higher dose of 500 mg of fulvestrant was found to be more effective than the 250 dose in the CONFIRM trial, showing a statistically significant improvement in PFS, leading to the FDA—approval of the higher dose of fulvestrant in 2010 [21]. A subsequent OS analysis showed a 19% reduction in risk of death and a 4.1 month advantage in median OS with the higher 500 of fulvestrant compared to the 250 mg dose [22]. The FIRST trial compared the 500 mg dose of fulvestrant to anastrozole and demonstrated a similar clinical benefit rate (73% vs. 67%), significantly longer median TTP of 23 versus 13 months and a significantly longer OS of 54 versus 48 months (although OS analysis was not planned in original protocol) [23–25]. The phase III, FALCON trial was recently reported in which 524 postmenopausal women were randomized to fulvestrant plus placebo versus anastrozole plus placebo. At a median follow-up of 25 months, PFS was prolonged with fulvestrant versus anastrozole (16.6 vs. 13.8 months; HR, 0.797; $P = 0.049$) [26]. Measures of quality of life and adverse events were similar between the two groups. These results suggest that fulvestrant could be acceptable as first-line therapy for metastatic disease in certain patients. When there are concerns regarding compliance and need for minimal toxicity due to age or comorbidities, fulvestrant could be considered earlier in the course of disease. The FALCON trial also recruited very pristine patients who had not been exposed to endocrine therapy, which may represent a small fraction of the breast cancer patient population.

Several studies have looked at the combination of fulvestrant and anastrozole in the first-line metastatic disease setting with discordant results. The FACT trial demonstrated no advantage to the combination of fulvestrant and anastrozole compared to anastrozole alone, whereas the SWOG trial (S02226) demonstrated an improvement in PFS of 15 months with the combination versus 13.5 months with anastrozole alone [27, 28]. Of note, all patients in the former trial received fulvestrant 250 mg, whereas in the latter trial a fraction received the higher dose of 500 mg. The discordant results may also be partially explained by the fact that a greater percentage of patients in the SWOG trial were completely endocrine therapy naïve compared to the FACT trial (60% vs. 30%).

The combination of fulvestrant and anastrozole was evaluated in the second-line setting in patients who had progressed on a non-steroidal AI. Patients in the SoFEA study were randomized to fulvestrant 250 mg plus anastrozole, fulvestrant 250 mg plus placebo, or exemestane alone. The combination of fulvestrant and an AI showed no improvement in PFS compared to the single arm options [29]. This study was limited by the use of the lower fulvestrant dose.

9.3 CDK 4/6 Inhibitors

While single-agent endocrine therapies have demonstrated modest benefit in the first and subsequent lines of therapy for women with ER-positive, MBC, combination therapy options have emerged as a more effective alternative for many patients. Growth of HR-positive breast cancer is dependent on cyclin-dependent kinases (CDK) 4 and 6 that promote progression from G1 to the S phase of the cell cycle. CDK inhibitors block the cyclin D1-CDK 4/6 complex, prevent RB protein phosphorylation, stop the cell cycle from progressing to the S phase, thereby preventing cancer cell proliferation.

The first CDK 4/6 inhibitor, palbociclib, received accelerated FDA approval in February 2015 based on phase II data from the PALOMA 1 trial [30]. This trial randomized women with no prior therapy for advanced breast cancer and no AI therapy within 12 months of randomization to letrozole alone or letrozole plus palbociclib. The combination therapy arm showed an improved PFS of 20.2 months compared to 10.2 months with letrozole alone (HR.49). The combination of letrozole and palbociclib was well-tolerated with neutropenia and leukopenia as the most common grade 3 and 4 adverse events. Fatigue, anemia, nausea, arthralgia, and alopecia were also reported.

PALOMA 2 was a randomized phase III study evaluating the same study population as in PALOMA 1. A total of 666 postmenopausal women with ER-positive MBC were randomized (2:1) between letrozole and palbociclib versus letrozole and placebo [31]. The combination therapy arm showed similar benefit to the phase II trial with a PFS of 24.7 months compared to 14.5 months in the single-agent letrozole arm (HR 0.58). There was a non-statistically significant improvement in OS.

The combination of palbociclib and fulvestrant was studied in the PALOMA 3 trial [32, 33]. A total of 521 patients with ER-positive, HER2-negative, advanced breast cancer who progressed on prior endocrine therapy or chemotherapy for advanced breast cancer, or within 12 months of completing adjuvant hormonal therapy, were randomized to fulvestrant alone or the combination of fulvestrant plus palbociclib. The combination resulted in an improvement in PFS from 4.6 months to 9.6 months (HR 0.46).

Multiple ongoing clinical trials are evaluating other potential indications for palbociclib and similar development plans are underway for other CDK 4/6 inhibitors. As an example, the PEARL study is evaluating palbociclib in combination with exemestane or fulvestrant compared to chemotherapy in patients previously treated with a non-steroidal AI or chemotherapy [34]. Another selective CDK 4/6 inhibitory, ribociclib, has also shown benefit when added to AI therapy. The MONALEESA 2 trial randomized 668 patients with HR-positive, HER2-negative, advanced breast cancer without prior systemic therapy for advanced disease to letrozole alone or letrozole plus ribociclib. At a median follow-up of 15.3 months, PFS was 63% in the combination arm and 42% in the single-agent letrozole arm [35]. Other clinical trials are ongoing with ribociclib in pre- and postmenopausal women, in the first- and second-line setting, and in combination with AIs, fulvestrant, or tamoxifen [36].

The CDK 4/6 inhibitor, abemaciclib, received breakthrough Therapy designation by the FDA in 2015. The MONARCH 1 study was a phase II study that evaluated 132 patients treated with abemaciclib monotherapy [37]. Patients had received a median of 3 lines of prior therapy including a median of 2 lines of chemotherapy for advanced breast cancer. Findings included an ORR of 17.4%, CBR 42.4%, PFS 6 months, and OS 17.7 months. MONARCH 2 is evaluating fulvestrant with or without abemaciclib in the first- and second-line setting [38]. MONARCH 3 is evaluating first-line therapy with abemaciclib in combination with anastrozole or letrozole [39].

9.4 mTOR Inhibitors

Resistance to endocrine therapy in breast cancer can be associated with activation of the mammalian target of rapamycin (mTOR) intracellular signaling pathway. Early studies showed that the mTOR inhibitor everolimus added to endocrine therapy improved antitumor activity. The BOLERO-2 study evaluated postmenopausal women with MBC who developed disease recurrence within 12 months of completion of adjuvant endocrine therapy, or within 1 month of treatment for advanced disease [40–42]. A total of 724 patients were randomized (2:1) to everolimus plus exemestane versus exemestane alone. Median PFS was 6.9 months in the combination arm versus 2.8 months in the single-agent exemestane arm. There was not a statistically significant overall survival benefit. The addition of everolimus is associated with increased toxicity, including mouth sores and rashes, compared to endocrine therapy alone. Ongoing studies are evaluating the addition of mTOR inhibitors to endocrine therapy in the adjuvant setting for patients with early stage, ER-positive breast cancer.

9.5 Resistance Mechanisms

Some cancers are refractory to estrogen-blocking therapies initially (*denovo* resistance), but more commonly, tumors become resistant to endocrine therapy as they are exposed to more, and different agents over time. Resistance to estrogen deprivation involves activation of growth factor pathways to bypass endocrine dependence. Mutations in the ESR1 ligand-binding domain have been demonstrated in hormone-resistant breast cancer. Somatic mutations of ESR1 have been found in <1% of primary breast cancers and in 19% of advanced breast cancers [43]. Acquisition of mutations increase with increasing tumor burden. In an analysis of ESR1 mutations by circulating tumor DNA in samples from the PALOMA 3 study, mutations were detected in 25% of baseline plasma samples [44]. Mutations were detected in 29% of patients treated with an AI, 2% of those treated with tamoxifen and 32% of those treated with tamoxifen and an AI. In the PALOMA 3 samples, mutations were neither prognostic nor predictive. Response rates were not significantly different between the ESR1-mutant and ESR1 wild-type patients. The addition of palbociclib offered similar benefit regardless of mutation status. In the SoFEA trial [28], patients were randomized to fulvestrant plus anastrozole or placebo versus exemestane. Interestingly, 39% of patients were found to have ESR1 mutations, and it was found that patients with ESR1 mutations treated with exemestane had a PFS of 2.6 months versus 5.7 months for those treated with fulvestrant (HR 0.52, $P = 0.02$) [45] ESR1 wild-type patients had no statistically significant difference in PFS when treated with exemestane versus fulvestrant. Within the exemestane group, patients with ESR1 mutations had worse PFS than those that were ESR1 wild-type. In this study, mutations were found to be both predictive and prognostic. The data from SoFEA provide early clinical evidence of the utility of ESR1 mutational status in selecting appropriate endocrine therapy.

Emerging data regarding mechanisms of endocrine resistance lead to several possible strategies for overcoming resistance. These include fulvestrant, combination therapies with CDK4/6 and mTOR inhibitors and other novel therapies in development to be discussed below. Therapies are also being developed to target the mutations in the estrogen receptor including some novel estrogen receptor downregulators with the ability to degrade mutant estrogen receptors.

9.6 PI3K Inhibitors

The PI3K/AKT/mTOR signaling pathway plays a critical role in mediating cell growth, survival, and angiogenesis. Mutations in this pathway are frequently seen in ER-positive breast cancer. Numerous agents are in development including PI3K inhibitors or agents that have multiple targets along the signaling pathway. The FERGI study evaluated fulvestrant versus fulvestrant plus the PI3Kinase inhibitor pictilisib in ER-positive, postmenopausal patients with advanced breast cancer and prior AI therapy. Combination therapy showed an improvement in PFS independent of PI3K mutation status [46]. The BELLE-2 study evaluated postmenopausal women with advanced breast cancer who progressed after AI, who were randomized to fulvestrant with or without the PI3K inhibitor buparsilib [47]. Combination therapy showed an improvement in PFS (6.9 vs. 5 months) with improvement observed in patients with PI3K mutations. BELLE-3 was presented at the 2016 San Antonio Breast Cancer Conference [48]. A total of 432 women who progressed after an AI and mTOR inhibitor were randomized in a 2:1 randomization to buparlisib plus fulvestrant versus fulvestrant alone. DFS was 3.9 months in the combination arm and 1.8 months in the single-agent arm. When stratified for PI3K mutation, a more significant difference of 4.2 versus 1.6 months was seen in the mutant group while no difference in PFS was seen in the wild-type group.

9.7 HDAC Inhibitors

Histone deacetylases are proteins required for control of gene expression and exert an anti-proliferative effect and promote apoptosis. Entinostat is a small molecule inhibitor of class I histone deacetylases. In the ENCORE 301 study, 130 patients who previously developed disease progression on an AI were randomized to treatment with exemestane plus entinostat versus exemestane alone. The combination showed an improved PFS of 4.3 versus 2.3 months in those receiving exemestane. Patients were heavily pretreated with 58% progressing on more than one endocrine agent and 62% having prior chemotherapy [49]. A phase 3 study is ongoing.

9.8 Summary—First-Line Endocrine Therapy for Advanced Breast Cancer

There are numerous first-line treatment options for postmenopausal women presenting with metastatic ER-positive breast cancer. Table 9.1 summarizes some of the landmark clinical trials in this setting, showing PFS ranging from 8 to 14 months with single-agent AI therapy to approximately 2 years with combination AI and palbociclib. Treatment recommendations vary based on several variables and can be stratified by women presenting with denovo metastatic disease or >12 months from completion of adjuvant endocrine therapy versus those presenting less than <12 months from completion of adjuvant endocrine therapy. Therapy also depends on whether the patient was treated with tamoxifen or an AI in the adjuvant setting and extent of disease at time of recurrence. Most women presenting without a visceral crisis can be treated with endocrine therapy.

For women with *denovo* metastatic disease or presenting >12 months from completion of adjuvant endocrine therapy, first-line endocrine options include tamoxifen, AI alone, AI plus palbociclib, fulvestrant or a combination of AI, and fulvestrant [4, 8–11, 16, 23–28, 30–32] Combination therapy with an AI and fulvestrant has been found to be most effective in patients without prior exposure to adjuvant endocrine therapy [28].

Patients with progression <12 months after completion of an AI in the adjuvant setting were not included in the PALOMA 1 and 2 studies. Treatment options for this population include a steroidal AI, tamoxifen, fulvestrant alone, or fulvestrant/palbociclib [33].

9.9 Summary—Second-Line Endocrine Therapy and Beyond

Sequential endocrine therapy is offered to most patients without rapid disease progression. Table 9.2 summarizes some of the significant clinical trials in the second-line metastatic setting, demonstrating PFS ranging from 3 to 6 months with single-agent therapy to 7–10 months with combination therapies. Treatment depends on what therapy was given in the first-line setting and the pace at which disease is progressing. Options include tamoxifen, AI alone, fulvestrant alone, fulvestrant plus palbociclib, or an AI plus everolimus [5–7, 17–19, 33, 40–42].

Table 9.1 Trials of first-line endocrine therapy for advanced breast cancer—PFS/TTP in months

Trial	Date	AI	Tam	Fulv 250 mg	Fulv 500 mg	Fulvestrant plus AI	AI plus CK4/6 inhibitor	Hazard ratio
Bonnetere et al. anastrozole vs. tamoxifen	2000	8.2	8.3					0.99
Nabholtz et al. anastrozole vs. tamoxifen	2000	11.1	5.6					0.81
Mouridsen et al. letrozole vs. tamoxifen	2003	9.4	6.0					0.72
Paridaens et al. exemestane vs. tamoxifen	2007	9.9	5.8					0.84
Howell et al. fulvestrant vs. tamoxifen	2004		8.3	6.8				1.18
FIRST Robertson et al. fulvestrant vs. anastrozole	2009	13			23			0.66
FACT Bergh et al. fulvestrant plus anastrozole vs. anastrozole	2012	10.2				10.8 (Fulv 250)		0.99
SWOG S02226 Mehta et al. fulv plus anastrozole vs. anastrozole	2012	13.5				15 (Fulv 250)		0.80
FALCON Robertson et al. fulvestrant 500 vs. anastrozole	2016	13.8				16.6 (Fulv 500)		0.80
PALOMA 2 Finnet al. letrozole plus palbociclib vs. letrozole	2015	14.6					24.7	0.58
MONALEESA[a] Hortobagyi et al. letrozole plus ribociclib vs. letrozole	2016	14.7					Not reached	0.56

[a]At a median follow-up of 15.3 months, PFS was 63% in the combination arm and 42% in the letrozole alone arm

Table 9.2 Trials of second-line endocrine therapy for advanced breast cancer—PFS/TTP in months

Trial	Date	AI	Tam	Fulv 250 mg	Fulv 500 mg	Fulv plus AI	CDK 4/6 inhibitor	mTOR inhibitor	Hazard ratio
Howell et al. fulvestrant vs. anastrozole	2002	5.1		5.5					0.98
EFFECT Chia et al. fulvestrant vs. exemestane[a]	2008	3.7		3.7					0.96
CONFIRM Di Leo et al. fulvestrant 250 vs. fulvestrant 500	2010			5.5	6.5				0.80
SoFEA Johnston et al. fulvestrant 250 vs fulvestrant plus anastrozole vs. exemestane	2013	3.4		4.8		4.4			1.00[b] 0.95[c]
PALOMA-3 Cristofanilli et al. fulvestrant plus palbo vs. fulvestrant	2016			4.6			9.6		0.46
BOLERO 2 Baselga et al. exemestane plus everolimus vs. everolimus	2012	2.8						6.9	0.43

[a]Approximately, 60% of patients had at least 2 prior endocrine therapies
[b]Fulvestrant plus anastrozole vs. fulvestrant plus placebo
[c]Fulvestrant plus placebo vs. exemestane

There is no proven difference between AIs in the second-line setting [13, 14]. Data have not shown a significant benefit to therapy with an AI plus fulvestrant in the second-line setting although studies are limited by the lower than standard dose of fulvestrant [29]. Tamoxifen has been shown to have a 10% ORR and CBR of 49% in the second-line setting with women previously treated with an AI [50].

For third-line therapy and beyond, decision making will again depend on extent of disease and presence or absence of symptomatic visceral disease and specific therapies used in earlier lines. Options include tamoxifen, AIs, fulvestrant, progestins, estrogen, androgens, combination therapies, and clinical trials with novel agents.

9.10 Conclusions

There has been much progress in the treatment of ER-positive MBC over the past 40 years. Single-agent therapy with tamoxifen, AIs and fulvestrant has been shown to be effective in numerous studies in the first-line setting and beyond. Combination regimens with CDK4/6 inhibitors and mTOR inhibitors have been shown to be superior to their monotherapy counterparts but with a modest increase in toxicities. Combination therapies can be beneficial in overcoming endocrine resistance, possibly delaying endocrine resistance, and therefore delaying the need for chemotherapy. Novel therapies such as PI3K inhibitors, HDAC inhibitors, and others in development are further expanding our therapeutic options in this patient population. In the future, ESR1 mutation status and other molecular markers will likely be used more frequently to guide therapy.

Specific treatment recommendations must take into account tumor biology, clinical features, and patient characteristics, and require a thoughtful conversation with patient weighing the benefits and toxicities of various therapeutic options.

References

1. Beatson G (1895) On the treatment of inoperable cases of carcinoma of the mamma-suggestions for a new method of treatment with illustrative cases. Lancet 2:104–107
2. Morgan LR Jr, Schein PS, Woolley PV et al (1976) Therapeutic use of tamoxifen in advanced cancer, correlation with biochemical parameters. Cancer Treat Rep 60:1437–1443
3. Rose C, Mouridsen HT (1984) Treatment of advanced breast cancer with tamoxifen. Recent Results Cancer Res 91:230–242
4. Muss HB, Case LD, Atkins JN et al (1994) Tamoxifen versus high dose oral medroxyprogesterone acetate as initial endocrine therapy for patients with metastatic breast cancer: a Piedmont Oncology Association study. J Clin Oncol 12:1630–1638
5. Buzdar A, Jonat W, Howell A et al (1996) Anastrozole, a potent and selective aromatase inhibitor versus megestrol acetate in postmenopausal women with advanced breast cancer: results of overview analysis of two phase III trials. Arimidex Study Group. J Clin Oncol 14:2000–2011
6. Kaufmann M, Bajetta E, Dirix LY et al (2000) Exemestane is superior to megestrol acetate after tamoxifen failure in postmenopausal women with advanced breast cancer: results of a phase III randomized double blind trial. The exemestane study group. J Clin Oncol 18:1399–1411
7. Budzar A, Douma J, Davidson N et al (2001) Phase III, multicenter, double-blind, randomized study of letrozole, an aromatase inhibitor, for advanced breast cancer versus megestrol acetate. J Clin Oncol 19:3357–3366
8. Bonneterre J, Thurlimann B, Robertson JF et al (2000) Anastrozole versus tamoxifen as first line therapy for advanced breast cancer in 668 postmenopausal women: results of the Tamoxifen or Arimidex Randomized Group Efficacy and Tolerability study. J Clin Oncol 18:3748–3757
9. Nabholtz JM, Budzar A, Pollak M et al (2000) Anastrozole is superior to tamoxifen as first-line therapy for advanced breast cancer in postmenopausal women: results of a North American Multicenter Randomized Trial. Arimidex Study Group. J Clin Oncol 18:3758–3767
10. Mouridsen H, Gershanovich M, Sun Y et al (2001) Superior efficacy of letrozole versus tamoxifen as first-line therapy for postmenopausal women with advanced breast cancer:

results of a phase III study of the International Letrozole Breast Cancer Group. J Clin Oncol 19:2596–2606

11. Paridaens R, Dirix L, Beex L et al (2008) Phase III study comparing exemestane with tamoxifen as first-line hormonal treatment of metastatic breast cancer in postmenopausal women: The European Organisation for Research and Treatment of Breast Cancer cooperative group. J Clin Oncol 28:4883–4890

12. Mauri D, Pavlidis N, Polyzos NP, Ionnidis JP (2006) Survival with aromatase inhibitors and inactivators versus standard hormonal therapy in advanced breast cancer: meta-analysis. J Natl Cancer Inst 98:1285–1299

13. Campos SM, Guastall JP, Subar M et al (2009) A Comparative study of exemestane versus anastrozole in patient with postmenopausal breast cancer with visceral metastases. Clin Breast Cancer 9:39–44

14. Rose C, Vtoraya O, Pluzanska A et al (2003) An open randomized trial of second line endocrine therapy in advanced breast cancer. Comparison of the aromatase inhibitors letrozole and anastrozole. Eur J Cancer 39:2318–2327

15. Wakeling AE, Dukes M, Bowler J (1991) A potent pure antiestrogen with clinical potential. Cancer Res 15:3867–3873

16. Howell A, Robertson JF, Abram P et al (2004) Comparison of fulvestrant versus tamoxifen for the treatment of advanced breast cancer in postmenopausal women previously untreated with endocrine therapy: a multinational, double-blind, randomized trial. J Clin Oncol 22:1605–1613

17. Howell A, Robertson JF, Quaresma Albano J et al (2002) Fulvestrant (ICI 182,780) is as effective as anastrozole in postmenopausal women with advanced breast cancer progressing after prior endocrine treatment. J Clin Oncol 20:3396–3403

18. Osborne CK, Pippen J, Jones SE et al (2002) A double-blind, randomized trial comparing the efficacy and tolerability of fulvestrant with anastrozole in postmenopausal women with advanced breast cancer progressing on prior endocrine therapy: results of a North American trial. J Clin Oncol 29:3386–3395

19. Chia S, Gradishar W, Mauriac J (2008) Double-blind randomized placebo controlled trial of fulvestrant compared with exemestane after prior nonsteroidal aromatase inhibitor therapy in postmenopausal women with hormone receptor positive advanced breast cancer: Results from EFFECT. J Clin Oncol 26:1664–1670

20. Howell A, Pippen J, Elledge RM (2005) Fulvestrant versus anastrozole for the treatment of advanced breast carcinoma: a prospective planned combined survival analysis of two multicenter trials. Cancer 104:236–239

21. Di Leo A, Jerusalem G, Petruzelka L et al (2010) Results of the CONFIRM phase III trial comparing fulvestrant 250 mg with fulvestrant 500 mg in postmenopausal women with estrogen receptor positive advanced breast cancer. J Clin Oncol 28:4594–4600

22. Di Leo A, Jerusalem G, Petruzelka L et al. (2014) Final overall survival: fulvestrant 500 vs 250 mg in the randomized CONFIRM trial. J Natl Cancer Inst 106: djt337

23. Robertson J, Llombart-Cussac A, Rolski J et al (2009) Activity of fulvestrant 500 mg versus anastrozole 1 mg as first-line treatment for advanced breast cancer: results from the FIRST study. J Clin Oncol 27:4530–4534

24. Robertson J, Lindemann J, Llombart-Cussac A et al (2012) Activity of fulvestrant 500 versus anastrozole 1 m as first-line treatment for advanced breast cancer-follow-up analysis from the randomized FIRST study. Breast Cancer Res Treat 136:503–511

25. Ellis M, Llombart-Cussac A, Feltl D et al (2015) Fulvestrant 500 mg versus anastrozole 1 mg for the first-line treatment of advanced breast cancer: overall survival analysis from the phase II FIRST study. J Clin Oncol 33:3781–3786

26. Robertson JF, Bondarenko I, Trishkina E et al (2016) Fulvestrant 500 mg versus anastrazole 1 mg for hormone receptor-positive advanced breast cancer (FALCON): an international, randomized, double-blind, phase 3 trial. Lancet 388:2997–3005

27. Bergh J, Jonsson PE, Lidbrink EK et al (2012) FACT: an open label randomized phase III study of fulvestrant and anastrozole in combination compared to anastrozole alone as first line therapy for patients with receptor-positive postmenopausal breast cancer. J Clin Oncol 30:1919–1925

28. Mehta RS, Barlow WE, Albain KS et al (2012) Combination anastrozole and fulvestrant in metastatic breast cancer. N Engl J Med 367:435–444

29. Johnstom SR, Kilburn LS, Ellis P et al (2013) Fulvestrant plus anastrozole or placebo versus exemestane alone after progression on non-steroidal aromatase inhibitors in postmenopausal patients with hormone-receptor positive locally advanced or metastatic breast cancer (SoFEA): a composite, multicenter, phase 3 randomised trial. Lancet Oncol 14:989–998

30. Finn RS, Crown JP, Lang I et al (2015) The cyclin-dependent kinase 4/6 inhibitor palbociclib in combination with letrozole versus letrozole alone as first-line treatment of estrogen receptor positive, HER-2 negative, advanced breast cancer (PALOMA-1/TRIO-18): a randomized phase 2 study. Lancet Oncol 16:25–35

31. Finn RS, Martin M, Rugo S (2016) Palbociclib and letrozole in advanced breast cancer. N Engl J Med 375:1925–1936

32. Turner NC, Ro J, Andre F et al (2015) Palbociclib in hormone receptor positive advanced breast cancer. N Engl J Med 373:209–219

33. Cristofanilli M, Turner NC, Bondarenko I et al (2016) Fulvestrant plus palbociclib versus fulvestrant plus placebo for treatment of hormone-receptor positive, HER2-negative metastatic breast cancer that progressed on previous endocrine therapy (PALOMA-3): final analysis of the multicenter, double blind, phase 3 randomised controlled trial. Lancet Oncol 17:425–439

34. Phase III Study of Palbociclib (PD-0332991) in Combination With Endocrine Therapy (Exemestane or Fulvestrant) Versus Chemotherapy (Capecitabine) in Hormonal Receptor (HR) Positive/HER2 Negative Metastatic Breast Cancer (MBC) Patients With Resistance to Non-steroidal Aromatase Inhibitors (PEARL) (ClinicalTrials.gov Identifier: NCT02028507)

35. Hortobagyi GN, Stemmer SM, Burris HA et al (2016) Ribociclib as First-Line Therapy for HR-positive, advanced breast cancer. N Engl J Med 375:1738–1748

36. A Randomized Double-blind, Placebo-controlled Study of Ribociclib in Combination With Fulvestrant for the Treatment of Men and Postmenopausal Women With Hormone Receptor Positive, HER2-negative, Advanced Breast Cancer Who Have Received no or Only One Line of Prior Endocrine Treatment MONALEESA 3 (ClinicalTrials.gov Identifier: NCT02422615)

37. Dickler MN, Tolaney SM, Rugo HS (2016) MONARCH 1: Results from a phase II study of abemaciclib, a CDK4 and CDK6 inhibitor, as monotherapy, in patients with HR +/ HER-2-breast cancer after chemotherapy for advanced disease. J Clin Oncol 34, suppl; abstr 510

38. MONARCH 2: A Randomized, Double-Blind, Placebo-Controlled, Phase 3 Study of Fulvestrant With or Without Abemaciclib, a CDK4/6 Inhibitor, for Women With Hormone Receptor Positive, HER2 Negative Locally Advanced or Metastatic Breast CancerA Study of Abemaciclib (LY2835219) ClinicalTrials.gov Identifier: NCT02107703

39. A Randomized, Double-Blind, Placebo-Controlled, Phase 3 Study of Nonsteroidal Aromatase Inhibitors (Anastrozole or Letrozole) Plus LY2835219, a CDK4/6 Inhibitor, or Placebo in Postmenopausal Women With Hormone Receptor-Positive, HER2-Negative Locoregionally Recurrent or Metastatic Breast Cancer With No Prior Systemic Therapy in This Disease Setting. A Study of Nonsteroidal Aromatase Inhibitors Plus Abemaciclib (LY2835219) in Postmenopausal Women With Breast Cancer (MONARCH 3) ClinicalTrials.gov Identifier: NCT02246621

40. Baselga J, Campone M, Piccart M et al (2012) Everolimus in postmenopausal hormone-receptor positive advanced breast cancer. N Engl J Med 366:520–529

41. Yardley DA, Noguchi S, Pritchard KI et al (2013) Everolimus plus exemestane in postmenopausal patients with HR-positive breast cancer: BOLERO-2 final progression free survival analysis. Adv Ther 30:870–884

42. Piccart M, Hortobagyi GN, Campone M (2014) Everolimus plus exemestane for hormone receptor positive, HER-2 negative advanced breast cancer: overall survival results from BOLERO-2. Ann Oncol 25:2357–2362

43. Toy W, Shen Y, Won H et al. (2013) ESR1 ligand binding domain mutations in hormone resistant breast cancer. Nat Genet 45: 1439–1445

44. Turner et al. (2016) Efficacy of palbociclib plus fulvestrant in patients with metastatic breast cancer and ESR1 mutations in circulating tumor DNA. J Clin Oncol 34 (suppl; abstr 512)

45. Fribbens C, O'Leary B, Kilburn L (2016) Plasma ESR1 mutations and the treatment of estrogen receptor-positive advanced breast cancer 34: 2961–2968

46. Krop I, Johnston S, Mayer IA (2014) The FERGI phase II study of the PI3 K inhibitor pictilisib (GDC-0941) plus fulvestrant vs fulvestrant plus placebo in patients with ER+, AI resistant advanced or metastatic breast cancer-Part I results. SABCS, Abstract S2-02

47. Baselga J, Im S-A, Iwata H et al. (2015) PIK3CA status in circulating tumor DNA predicts efficacy of buparlisib plus fulvestrant in postmenopausal women with endocrine-resistant HER+/HER2− advanced breast cancer: first results from the randomized, phase III BELLE-2 trial. SABCS, Abstract S6-01

48. Di Leo A, Lee K, Ciuelos E et al. (2016) BELLE-3: a phase III study of buparlisib and fulvestrant in postmenopausal women with HR+, HER2-, AI-treated, locally advanced or metastatic breast cancer, who progressed on or after mTOR inhibitor-based treatment. SABCS, Abstract S4-07

49. Yardley DA, Ismail-Khan R, Klein P (2011) Results of ENCORE 301, a randomized phase II, double blind, placebo controlled study of exemestane with or without entinostat in postmenopausal women with locally recurrent or metastatic estrogen receptor positive breast cancer progressing on a nonsteroidal AI. J Clin Oncol suppl 27, abstr 268

50. Thurlimann B, Robertson JF, Nabholtz JM et al (2003) Efficacy of tamoxifen following anastrozole compared to anastrozole following tamoxifen as first-line treatment for advanced breast cancer in postmenopausal women. Eur J Cancer 39:2310

Immune Checkpoint Blockade for Breast Cancer

10

April Swoboda and Rita Nanda

Contents

Abstract

An effective antitumor immune response requires interaction between cells of the adaptive and innate immune system. Three key elements are required: generation of activated tumor-directed T cells, infiltration of activated T cells into the tumor microenvironment, and killing of tumor cells by activated T cells. Tumor immune evasion can occur as a result of the disruption of each of these three key T cell activities, resulting in three distinct cancer-immune phenotypes. The immune inflamed phenotype, characterized by the presence of a robust tumor immune infiltrate, suggests impaired activated T cell killing of tumor cells related to the presence of inhibitory factors. Programmed death receptor-1 (PD-1) is an inhibitory transmembrane protein expressed on T cells, B cells, and NK cells. The interaction between PD-1 and its ligands (PD-L1/L2) functions as

A. Swoboda · R. Nanda (✉)
Section of Hematology/Oncology, 5841 S. Maryland Ave, MC 2115, Chicago,
IL 60616, USA
e-mail: rnanda@medicine.bsd.uchicago.edu

© Springer International Publishing AG 2018
W. J. Gradishar (ed.), *Optimizing Breast Cancer Management*, Cancer Treatment
and Research 173, https://doi.org/10.1007/978-3-319-70197-4_10

an immune checkpoint against unrestrained cytotoxic T effector cell activity—it promotes peripheral T effector cell exhaustion and conversion of T effector cells to immunosuppressive T regulatory (Treg) cells. Immune checkpoint inhibitors, which block the PD-1/PD-L1 axis and reactivate cytotoxic T effector cell function, are actively being investigated for the treatment of breast cancer.

Keywords
Breast cancer · Immunotherapy · Immune checkpoint inhibitors

10.1 Introduction

The immune system is controlled by a delicate balance of factors that work to both initiate immune responses and inhibit excessive inflammation induced by immunity. Cells from both the innate and adaptive immune systems work to eradicate pathogens and other threats, including tumors. Early in tumorigenesis, an acute inflammatory response is triggered, leading to the recruitment of effectors of innate immunity, including macrophages, natural killer (NK) cells, and dendritic cells, resulting in the generation of interferon (IFN) gamma and interleukin-12. These factors stimulate tumor cell killing via macrophages and NK cells. Simultaneously, dendritic cells mature, process tumor-associated antigens, and present these antigens to naïve T cells. These T cells in turn become activated and travel to and infiltrate the tumor microenvironment, where they work to eradicate tumor cells. This adaptive immune response can result in either the complete eradication of a tumor or the selection of tumor cells which evade immune surveillance.

For an effective antitumor immune response, three key elements are required: generation of activated tumor-directed T cells, infiltration of activated T cells into the tumor microenvironment, and killing of tumor cells by activated T cells [1]. Tumor immune evasion can occur as a result of the disruption of each of these three key T cell activities, resulting in three distinct cancer-immune phenotypes [2]. The immune desert phenotype—characterized by the absence of tumor-infiltrating immune cells—is generally seen when there is impaired T cell generation, related to immunologic ignorance, tolerance, or failure of T cell priming and activation. The immune excluded phenotype is characterized by the inability of T cells to infiltrate the tumor microenvironment and is likely related to the expression of immune suppressive cytokines or to barriers of infiltration into the tumor bed. The immune inflamed phenotype, characterized by the presence of a robust tumor immune infiltrate, suggests an arrest in the antitumor immune response related to the presence of inhibitory factors. By characterizing the biology of these different phenotypes, underlying immune escape mechanisms can be identified and strategies to activate antitumor immune responses that will lead to effective and sustained tumor eradication can be developed.

Immune checkpoint inhibition has emerged as an effective treatment for a variety of malignancies, with FDA approvals for new indications occurring at a rapid pace. The study of immunotherapy in breast cancer has been relatively delayed compared to other malignancies, because until recently breast cancer was not thought to be an immunogenic disease. We now know that many breast cancers are immunogenic and are enriched in tumor-infiltrating lymphocytes (TILs) [3]. Reactivating the immune system to eradicate breast cancers has emerged as a promising treatment strategy, and immune checkpoint inhibition has demonstrated activity in both advanced and early stage breast cancer. This chapter provides an overview of breast cancer immunobiology and immune-based treatment strategies for breast cancer.

10.2   Rationale for Immunotherapy for Breast Cancer

Breast cancer has historically been viewed as immunologically silent. However, a number of observations over the last several years have suggested that at least a subset of breast cancers is capable of stimulating the immune system. It has long been observed that some breast tumors have a substantial lymphocytic infiltration [4]. These lymphocyte predominant breast cancers are characterized by a dense lymphocytic infiltration, with tumor-infiltrating immune (TILs) cells comprising 50% or more of the tumor bed. A number of studies have demonstrated that the higher the proportion of TILs, the more favorable the prognosis. In an analysis of almost 16,000 patients, the presence of TILs at diagnosis was prognostic of outcome in patients with TNBC and HER2-positive breast cancers [5]. In a study of 481 patients with TNBC, there was a 14% improvement in disease-free survival for each 10% increase in TILs [6]. In a series of 387 HER2-positive breast cancer patients, TILs were inversely correlated with recurrence, with each 1% increase in the proportion of TILs correlating with a 3% reduction in the risk of recurrence [7]. TIL density, however, does not appear to be prognostic of outcome in ER-positive disease [8]. In addition to being prognostic in some breast cancer subtypes, TILs appear to be predictive of response to therapy. Two studies demonstrated a correlation between TIL density and improved outcome with anthracycline-based therapy [9]. Outcomes of HER2-positive breast cancers treated with trastuzumab-based therapies, however, show differing results. The FinHER study demonstrated an improved outcome with increased TIL density, while the opposite was observed in the NCCTG N9831 trial [10, 11].

Programmed death receptor-1 (PD-1) is an inhibitory transmembrane protein expressed on T cells, B cells, and NK cells. Its ligands are programmed death-ligand 1 (PD-L1), also known as B7-H1, and programmed death-ligand 2 (PD-L2), also known as B7-H2 [12]. PD-L1 is expressed on the surface of multiple types of cells, including tumor and hematopoietic cells, while PD-L2 is primarily expressed on hematopoietic cells. The interaction between PD-1 and its ligands directly inhibits apoptosis of tumor cells, promotes peripheral T effector cell exhaustion, and promotes conversion of T effector cells to immunosuppressive T regulatory (Treg) cells. PD-1 and PD-L1/L2 are upregulated in the context of pro-effector cytokines (such as IFN-gamma) secreted by CD8+ TILs, highlighting their role as immune checkpoints—they function as a physiologic "brake" on unrestrained cytotoxic T effector function. PD-L1 is expressed by approximately 20% of breast cancers, with TNBC and HER2-positive breast cancers expressing higher levels of expression than ER-positive breast cancers (33, 56 and 11%, respectively). The prognostic value of PD-L1 expression has been evaluated, and while some studies suggest PD-L1 expression is associated with a more favorable prognosis, others suggest that expression is associated with a poor prognosis. While the prognostic significance of PD-L1 expression in breast cancer remains unclear, the greater likelihood of response to PD-1 and PD-L1 blockade in PD-L1 positive cancers led to the interest in investigating immune checkpoint inhibitors for breast cancer.

10.3 PD-1 Blockade

Pembrolizumab (MK-3475) is a highly selective, humanized immunoglobulin (Ig) G4-κ monoclonal antibody specific for PD-1, currently FDA-approved for use in advanced melanoma, non-small cell lung cancer, squamous cell carcinoma of the head and neck (SCCHN), urothelial carcinoma, and classical Hodgkin lymphoma. In May 2017, it received accelerated approval for adult and pediatric patients with unresectable or metastatic microsatellite instability-high (MSI-H) or mismatch repair deficient (dMMR) solid tumors that have progressed following prior treatment and who have no satisfactory alternative treatment options. This approval marks the first tumor tissue/site-agnostic indication granted by the FDA, with approval based on a common biomarker rather than the location of the body where the tumor originated. Pembrolizumab has been studied in breast cancer both as monotherapy and in combination with chemotherapy, for both advanced and early stage breast cancer.

KEYNOTE-012 was a phase Ib multicohort study of single agent pembrolizumab in patients with advanced PD-L1-positive (PD-L1+) solid tumors, including TNBC, gastric cancer, urothelial cancer, and head and neck cancer [13]. PD-L1 positivity was defined as PD-L1 expression in stroma or $\geq 1\%$ of tumor cells by immunohistochemistry (IHC) using the Merck 22C3 antibody. The TNBC cohort enrolled 32 women with recurrent or metastatic PD-L1+ TNBC; of the 111 patients screened for PD-L1 expression, 58.6% had PD-L1+ tumors. Median age was 50.5 years in this heavily pretreated population; patients had received a median of two prior lines of systemic therapy for metastatic disease, with 46.9% of patients having received ≥ 3 lines of therapy. Among the 27 patients who were evaluable for antitumor activity, the primary endpoint of objective response rate [ORR; defined as complete responses (CR) plus partial responses (PR)] was 18.5% (1 CR, 4 PR), with a median time to response of 17.9 weeks (range 7.3–32.4 weeks). Durable responses were observed, with the median duration of response not yet reached (range 15.0 to ≥ 47.3 weeks), including three responders remaining on treatment for over 1 year. Treatment-related adverse events (TRAEs) were mild and similar to those observed in other tumor types; most common were arthralgias, fatigue, myalgias, and nausea. Five patients (15.6%) had grade ≥ 3 AEs, and there was one on treatment death due to disseminated intravascular coagulation (DIC).

The phase II KEYNOTE-086 study evaluated pembrolizumab monotherapy in two cohorts: previously treated metastatic TNBC (mTNBC) regardless of PD-L1 expression (Cohort A) and first-line PD-L1+ mTNBC (Cohort B) [14, 15]. Of the 170 patients enrolled in cohort A, (median age 53.5 years; range, 28–85 years), 43.5% had ≥ 3 prior lines of therapy and 61.8% had PD-L1+ tumors [14]. After a median follow-up of 10.9 months, 9 patients (5.3%) remained on pembrolizumab. Primary endpoint of overall ORR was 4.7% (95% CI, 2.3–9.2%); ORR was the same regardless PD-L1 expression (4.8% in PD-L1+ patients vs. 4.7% in PD-L1-negative patients). Disease control rate was 7.6% (DCR = CR + PR + stable disease [SD] ≥ 24 weeks; 95% CI, 4.4–12.7 weeks). Median duration of response (DOR) was 6.3 months (range 1.2+ to 10.3+ months); median progression-free survival (PFS) and overal survival (OS) were 2.0 months (95% CI 1.9–2.0) and 8.9 months (95% CI 7.2–11.2 months), respectively. TRAEs of any grade and grade ≥ 3 occurred in 60 and 12.4% of patients, respectively. There were no deaths due to AE and 4% of patients discontinued pembrolizumab due to TRAEs. Of the first 52 patients enrolled to cohort B of KEYNOTE-086 for first-line treatment of PD-L1+ mTNBC, median age was 53 years (range, 26–80 years), and 87% had received prior (neo)adjuvant therapy [16]. At median follow-up of 7.0 months (range 4.4–12.5 months), 15 (29%) patients remained on pembrolizumab. The primary endpoint was safety; TRAEs occurred in 37 (71%) patients and the most common were fatigue (31%), nausea (15%), and diarrhea (13%). Four (8%) patients experienced grade ≥ 3 TRAEs: back pain, fatigue, hyponatremia, hypotension, and migraine ($n = 1$ each). No patients died or discontinued pembrolizumab due to an AE. The ORR was 23.1% (95% CI 14–36%), with 2 CRs and 10 PRs. The median time to response was 8.7 weeks (range 8.1–17.7 weeks) and median DOR was 8.4 months (range, 2.1+ to 8.4 months), with 8 (67%) responses ongoing at data cutoff. The median PFS was 2.1 months (95% CI, 2.0–3.9 months), with estimated 6-month PFS rate 28%. A randomized phase III trial of pembrolizumab monotherapy versus chemotherapy in metastatic TNBC, KEYNOTE-119, is ongoing [17].

The phase Ib KEYNOTE-028 trial examined pembrolizumab in 25 patients with metastatic PD-L1+ ER+/HER2-negative breast cancer [18]. A total of 261 patients were screened, and 18.4% had PD-L1+ disease. The median age was 53 years (range, 36–79 years), and 80% of patients had received ≥ 3 prior lines of therapy for advanced disease. The overall response rate was 12% (95% CI, 2.5–31.2%), consisting of 3 PRs. Four patients (16%; 95% CI, 4.5–36.1%) had SD, and the clinical benefit rate (CBR; defined as ORR plus SD for ≥ 24 weeks) was 20%. The median time to response was 8 weeks, and all 3 responders remained on study treatment at the time of initial presentation at the 2015 San Antonio Breast Cancer Symposium (SABCS). TRAEs included arthralgia, fatigue, myalgia, and nausea, and were mostly grade 1-2. Grade ≥ 3 TRAEs included autoimmune hepatitis, increased gamma-glutamyl transferase (GGT) levels, muscle weakness, nausea, and septic shock; there were no treatment-related deaths.

A phase Ib/II study evaluated pembrolizumab in combination with eribulin in patients with mTNBC unselected for PD-L1 expression [19]. An interim analysis of the first 39 enrolled patients ($n = 7$, phase Ib; $n = 32$, phase II) was presented at the 2016 SABCS. The median age of participants was 53 years (range, 32–80 years) and the study included patients previously treated with 0–2 lines of chemotherapy in the metastatic setting. Primary endpoints were determination of safety and tolerability (phase Ib) and evaluation of ORR (phase II); secondary endpoints included evaluation of PFS, OS, and DOR. No dose-limiting toxicities (DLTs) were observed in phase Ib. The most common TRAEs were fatigue, nausea, peripheral neuropathy, neutropenia, and alopecia, with the most frequent grade ≥ 3 AEs being neutropenia and fatigue, side effects frequently observed with eribulin monotherapy. The overall ORR was 33.3% (1 CR, 12 PR). In stratum 1, which consisted of patients that were previously untreated in the metastatic setting, the ORR was 41.2% (95% CI, 19.3–62.8%) versus 27.3% (95% CI, 11.3–46.4%) in stratum 2 (1-2 prior lines of treatment). PD-L1 status did not predict response to treatment: ORR was 29.4% (95% CI, 11.1–51.1%) in the PD-L1+ patients versus 33.3% (95% CI, 14.1–54.6%) in PD-L1− patients. Overall, the combination of pembrolizumab and eribulin demonstrated activity in mTNBC, and AEs observed with the combination were comparable to those observed historically with either treatment as monotherapy. A two-arm phase III clinical trial, KEYNOTE-355, to evaluate the safety and efficacy of pembrolizumab in combination with three different chemotherapies (paclitaxel, nab-paclitaxel, carboplatin/gemcitabine) in the first-line treatment of mTNBC is currently underway (ClinicalTrials.gov identifier: NCT02819518).

I-SPY2 (Investigation of Serial Studies to Predict Your Therapeutic Response With Imaging And molecular Analysis 2) is an ongoing phase II platform trial in patients with stage II-III breast cancer that is evaluating multiple novel therapies in combination with standard neoadjuvant chemotherapy (NACT) with paclitaxel followed by doxorubicin/cyclophosphamide [20]. The I-SPY2 trial utilizes a novel adaptive randomization algorithm, based on biomarker "signatures," to assign patients to treatment arms that are performing well for patients who share their biomarker signature. The primary endpoint for I-SPY2 is pathologic complete response rate (pCR rate) defined as TNM stage ypT0/TisN0. In 69 patients, the addition of 4 cycles of pembrolizumab administered concurrently with paclitaxel significantly increased the estimated pCR rates. The estimated pCR rates in the TNBC population were 60% in the pembrolizumab group (95% Bayesian probability interval [PI], 43–78%) versus 20% (95% PI, 6–33%) in the control group of standard NACT alone. In patients with hormone receptor-positive (HR+)/HER2-negative breast cancer, the estimated pCR rate was 34% (95% PI, 19–48%) in the pembrolizumab arm versus 13% (95% PI, 3–24%) in the control arm. In the pembrolizumab arm, there were seven grade ≥ 3 immune-related adverse events (IRAEs): adrenal insufficiency ($n = 6$, includes primary and secondary adrenal insufficiency (AI) and colitis ($n = 1$). Five of those diagnosed with adrenal insufficiency presented after completion of AC (10–12 weeks after last pembrolizumab dose), and one presented prior to AC (5 weeks after first pembrolizumab dose). Eight patients had grade 1–2 thyroid abnormalities. Due to the toxicities observed, serial screening AM cortisol levels have been incorporated into the trial, in addition to ongoing serial thyroid function testing. The most common grade ≥ 3 AEs in the pembrolizumab arm were diarrhea, febrile neutropenia, fatigue, anemia, and nausea. Based on Bayesian predictive probability of success in a confirmatory phase III trial, pembrolizumab "graduated" from the I-SPY2 trial for all signatures in which it was tested (TNBC, all HER2-negative, and HR+/HER2-negative). Of note, this is the first investigational agent in the trial to graduate in the HR+/HER2-negative signature.

The phase III KEYNOTE-522 study is an ongoing neoadjuvant trial evaluating the combination of carboplatin/paclitaxel with or without pembrolizumab followed by doxorubicin/cyclophosphamide with or without pembrolizumab in patients with TNBC (ClinicalTrials.gov identifier: NCT03036488). Primary endpoints are pCR (defined as ypT0/TisN0) and event-free survival (EFS). In the adjuvant setting, Southwest Oncology Group (SWOG) S1418 is an ongoing phase III clinical trial that seeks to define the role of pembrolizumab in patients with TNBC that have residual disease after NACT; patients are randomized to either adjuvant pembrolizumab or placebo for 1 year (ClinicalTrials.gov identifier: NCT02954874).

In HER2+ disease, both trastuzumab and ado-trastuzumab emtansine (T-DM1) have been shown to increase TILs, suggesting that untreated HER2 signaling could be a mechanism of immune suppression [21, 22]. Multiple studies are investigating the combination of anti-HER2 therapy with immune checkpoint inhibitors. PANACEA is a phase Ib/II trial evaluating the safety and efficacy of pembrolizumab and trastuzumab in trastuzumab-resistant, PD-L1+ HER2+ metastatic breast cancer [23]. PembroMab is a phase Ib/II trial evaluating the safety and efficacy of pembrolizumab and trastuzumab or ado-trastuzumab emtansine in patients with metastatic HER2+ breast cancer, regardless of PD-L1 status (ClinicalTrials.gov identifier: NCT02318901).

10.4 PD-L1 Blockade

Atezolizumab (MPDL3280A) is a high-affinity, engineered, fully human IgG_1 monoclonal antibody that inhibits the interaction of PD-L1 with PD-1 and B7.1 (CD80), both of which are negative regulators of T-lymphocyte activation [24]. Because PD-L1 is expressed on activated T cells, atezolizumab was engineered with a modification in the Fc domain that eliminates antibody-dependent cellular cytotoxicity (ADCC) at clinically relevant doses, thus preventing the depletion of T cells expressing PD-L1 [25]. It is currently FDA-approved for a number of advanced cancers, including urothelial carcinoma and non-small cell lung cancer.

A phase Ia study evaluated the safety and efficacy of atezolizumab monotherapy in multiple disease-specific cohorts, including a cohort of 115 mTNBC patients [26]. The TNBC cohort initially enrolled patients with PD-L1+ disease, but was later amended to include patients with PD-L1-negative disease. Among pre-screened patients, 63% had PD-L1+ tumors, defined as containing $\geq 5\%$ PD-L1+ tumor-infiltrating lymphocytes (TILs) using the SP142 antibody. Median age was 53 years (range, 29–82 years) and the population was heavily pretreated, with 58% of patients having received ≥ 3 systemic therapies in the metastatic setting. ORR in the 112 evaluable patients was 10% (95% CI, 5–17%), with median DOR 21.1 months (range, 2.8–26.5+ months) and median PFS 1.4 months (95% CI, 1.3–1.6 months). Three patients initially classified as having PD appear to have had pseudoprogression, with evidence of ongoing clinical benefit and durable regression of target lesions despite the appearance of new lesions [27]. There was a marked difference in ORR depending on the line of treatment; ORR in patients previously untreated for metastatic disease was 26% (95% CI, 9–51%), compared to 4% in the second-line setting (95% CI, 0–18%), and 8% in patients who had received three or more lines of therapy (95% CI, 3–17%). The median OS at a median follow-up of 15.2 months was 9.3 months (95% CI, 7.0–12.6 months). The OS rate was 41% at 1 year (95% CI, 31–51%) and 22% at both 2 and 3 years (95% CI 12–32%). Remarkably, OS for the 11 patients with an objective response (CR or PR) was 100% at 2 years. TRAEs were frequent (observed in 63% of patients); the most common were pyrexia, fatigue, and nausea, which were typically grade 1-2 and easily managed. Eleven percent of patients experienced grade ≥ 3 TRAEs, and there were two treatment-related deaths as assessed by the investigators (pulmonary hypertension and death not otherwise specified in a hospitalized patient). Exploratory biomarker analyses suggested that higher levels of TILs, and to a lesser extent PD-L1 positivity, are associated with a longer overall survival with atezolizumab monotherapy.

The combination of atezolizumab and nab-paclitaxel was evaluated for safety and clinical activity in a phase Ib study of patients with mTNBC unselected for PD-L1 expression [28]. Thirty-two patients were enrolled; median age was 55.5 years (range, 32–84 years), and patients could have received 0–3 prior lines of therapy. At time of data cutoff, confirmed ORR was 38% (95% CI, 21–56%) in the 32 patients evaluable for efficacy. Two additional patients had pseudoprogression; they developed new lesions and were scored as PD based on RECIST (Response Evaluation Criteria in Solid Tumors), but had partial responses in target lesions and remained on treatment with prolonged biologic response. In the PD-L1+ cohort, ORR was 36% (95% CI, 11–69%) compared to 30% (95% CI, 7–65%) in the PD-L1-negative cohort. Grade 3 or 4 hematologic AEs was observed in 56% of patients; however, these were manageable and did not require treatment discontinuation. No DLT or treatment-related deaths occurred. Based on these results, the combination of atezolizumab and nab-paclitaxel is currently being investigated in the IMpassion 130 trial, a phase III randomized, double-blind, placebo-controlled study for the first-line treatment of patients with mTNBC [29]. The phase III NeoTRIPaPDL1 study is evaluating the combination of nab-paclitaxel and carboplatin with or without atezolizumab for patients with locally advanced TNBC in the neoadjuvant setting; primary endpoint is EFS (ClinicalTrials.gov identifier: NCT02620280). A single arm, phase II clinical trial assessing the safety and efficacy of atezolizumab in combination with paclitaxel, trastuzumab, and pertuzumab in patients with locally advanced, unresectable, or metastatic HER2+ breast cancer has recently started enrolling patients (ClinicalTrials.gov identifier: NCT03125928).

Avelumab (MSB0010718C) is a fully human anti-PD-L1 $IgG_1-\kappa$ monoclonal antibody that is currently FDA-approved for advanced urothelial carcinoma and Merkel cell carcinoma. In the phase Ib JAVELIN solid tumor trial, avelumab was investigated in locally advanced or metastatic breast cancer refractory to standard of care therapy [30]. Patients were unselected for PD-L1 expression or breast cancer subtype. A total of 168 patients were enrolled, with median age 55 years (range, 31–81 years). The population was heavily pretreated, with 52.4% of patients having had ≥ 3 prior lines of therapy. Fifty-eight of 168 patients (34.5%) had TNBC; 43% had HR+/HER2-negative disease; 15.5% had HER2+ disease; and 7% had disease of unknown molecular subtype. The ORR for the entire cohort was 4.8% (95% CI, 2.1–9.2%), with 1 CR and 7 PR; 5 of the 8 responses were ongoing at the time of data cutoff. Stable disease was observed in 39 patients (23.2%) for an overall DCR of 28%. In the TNBC subgroup ($n = 58$), there were 5 PRs for an ORR of 8.6% (95% CI, 2.9–19.0%). In contrast, the response rates in the HR+/HER2-negative ($n = 72$) and HER2+ ($n = 26$) cohorts were 2.8% (95% CI, 0.3–9.7%) and 3.8% (95% CI, 0.1–19.6%), respectively. Among TNBC patients with $\geq 10\%$ PD-L1 + immune cells within the tumor, so-called immune cell "hotspots," 44.4% (4 of 9) had a response to therapy (PR). TRAEs were observed in 71.4% of patients; the most common were fatigue, nausea, and infusion-related reactions. Grade ≥ 3 TRAEs occurred in 14.3% of patients, and included fatigue, anemia, increased GGT, autoimmune hepatitis, and arthralgias. There were two treatment-related deaths (acute liver failure and respiratory distress).

10.5 Conclusions

A subset of breast cancer is clearly immunogenic. The observations that some tumors are characterized by dense lymphocytic infiltration and expression of PD-L1 led to the investigation of immune checkpoint inhibition in advanced breast cancer. Immune checkpoint inhibition has demonstrated modest single agent activity in advanced breast cancer. While overall response rates are relatively low, the responses observed are remarkably durable, and therapy is well tolerated with mild and easily manageable side effects. Response correlates with TIL density, and the highest response rates have been observed in TNBC, particularly in the frontline setting. PD-L1-positivity enriches for responders, but is not a consistent predictor of response. Initial studies of immune checkpoint inhibitors in combination with chemotherapy for early stage disease have demonstrated promising efficacy, but also an increased incidence of immune-related toxicity. While treatment with immune checkpoint inhibitors clearly benefits subsets of patients, more precise biomarkers of response are needed, as well as strategies to increase response rates. A number of randomized phase II and III clinical trials of PD-1/PD-L1 inhibitors in combination with chemotherapy, targeted therapies, radiotherapy, and other immune checkpoint inhibitors are underway, and based on the promising results observed to date, immune checkpoint inhibitors are likely to gain regulatory approval for breast cancer in the near future.

References

1. Chen DS, Mellman I (2013) Oncology meets immunology: the cancer-immunity cycle. Immunity 39(1):1–10
2. Chen DS, Mellman I (2017) Elements of cancer immunity and the cancer-immune set point. Nature 541(7637):321–330
3. Cimino-Mathews A et al (2016) PD-L1 (B7-H1) expression and the immune tumor microenvironment in primary and metastatic breast carcinomas. Hum Pathol 47(1):52–63
4. Loi S et al (2013) Prognostic and predictive value of tumor-infiltrating lymphocytes in a phase III randomized adjuvant breast cancer trial in node-positive breast cancer comparing the addition of docetaxel to doxorubicin with doxorubicin-based chemotherapy: BIG 02-98. J Clin Oncol 31(7):860–867
5. Savas P et al (2016) Clinical relevance of host immunity in breast cancer: from TILs to the clinic. Nat Rev Clin Oncol 13(4):228–241
6. Adams S et al (2014) Prognostic value of tumor-infiltrating lymphocytes in triple-negative breast cancers from two phase III randomized adjuvant breast cancer trials: ECOG 2197 and ECOG 1199. J Clin Oncol 32(27):2959–2966
7. Salgado R et al (2015) Tumor-infiltrating lymphocytes and associations with pathological complete response and event-free survival in her2-positive early-stage breast cancer treated with lapatinib and trastuzumab: a secondary analysis of the NeoALTTO trial. JAMA Oncol 1 (4):448–454
8. Ali HR et al (2014) Association between CD8+ T-cell infiltration and breast cancer survival in 12,439 patients. Ann Oncol 25(8):1536–1543
9. Dieci MV et al (2015) Prognostic and predictive value of tumor-infiltrating lymphocytes in two phase III randomized adjuvant breast cancer trials. Ann Oncol 26(8):1698–1704
10. Perez EA et al (2016) Association of stromal tumor-infiltrating lymphocytes with recurrence-free survival in the N9831 adjuvant trial in patients with early-stage HER2-positive breast cancer. JAMA Oncol 2(1):56–64
11. Loi S et al (2014) Tumor infiltrating lymphocytes are prognostic in triple negative breast cancer and predictive for trastuzumab benefit in early breast cancer: results from the FinHER trial. Ann Oncol 25(8):1544–1550
12. Freeman GJ et al (2000) Engagement of the PD-1 immunoinhibitory receptor by a novel B7 family member leads to negative regulation of lymphocyte activation. J Exp Med 192 (7):1027–1034
13. Nanda R et al (2016) Pembrolizumab in patients with advanced triple-negative breast cancer: phase Ib KEYNOTE-012 study. J Clin Oncol 34(21):2460–2467
14. Adams S et al (2017) Phase 2 study of pembrolizumab (pembro) monotherapy for previously treated metastatic triple-negative breast cancer (mTNBC): KEYNOTE-086 cohort A. J Clin Oncol 35(15_suppl):1008
15. Adams S et al (2017) Phase 2 study of pembrolizumab as first-line therapy for PD-L1, Äipositive metastatic triple-negative breast cancer (mTNBC): Preliminary data from KEYNOTE-086 cohort B. J Clin Oncol 35(15_suppl):1088

16. Adams S et al (2017) Phase 2 study of pembrolizumab as first-line therapy for PD-L1–positive metastatic triple-negative breast cancer (mTNBC): Preliminary data from KEYNOTE-086 cohort B. J Clin Oncol 35(15_suppl):1088

17. Winer EP et al (2016) KEYNOTE-119: A randomized phase III study of single-agent pembrolizumab (MK-3475) vs single-agent chemotherapy per physician's choice for metastatic triple-negative breast cancer (mTNBC). J Clin Oncol 34(15_suppl): p. TPS1102-TPS1102

18. Rugo H et al (2016) Abstract S5-07: Preliminary efficacy and safety of pembrolizumab (MK-3475) in patients with PD-L1–positive, estrogen receptor-positive (ER+)/HER2-negative advanced breast cancer enrolled in KEYNOTE-028. Cancer Res 76(4 suppl): p. S5-07-S5-07

19. Tolaney S et al (2017) Abstract P5-15-02: Phase 1b/2 study to evaluate eribulin mesylate in combination with pembrolizumab in patients with metastatic triple-negative breast cancer. Cancer Res 77(4 suppl): p. P5-15-02-P5-15-02

20. Nanda R et al (2017) Pembrolizumab plus standard neoadjuvant therapy for high-risk breast cancer (BC): Results from I-SPY 2. J Clin Oncol 35(15 suppl):506

21. Gennari R et al (2004) Pilot study of the mechanism of action of preoperative trastuzumab in patients with primary operable breast tumors overexpressing HER2. Clin Cancer Res 10(17):5650–5655

22. Muller P et al (2015) Trastuzumab emtansine (T-DM1) renders HER2+ breast cancer highly susceptible to CTLA-4/PD-1 blockade. Sci Transl Med 7(315): pp 315ra188

23. Loi S et al (2016) Abstract OT3-01-05: PANACEA (IBCSG 45-13/BIG 4-13): A phase Ib/II trial evaluating the efficacy of pembrolizumab and trastuzumab in patients with trastuzumab-resistant, HER2-positive, metastatic breast cancer. Cancer Res 76(4 suppl): p. OT3-01-05-OT3-01-05

24. Herbst RS et al (2014) Predictive correlates of response to the anti-PD-L1 antibody MPDL3280A in cancer patients. Nature 515(7528):563–567

25. Powles T et al (2014) MPDL3280A (anti-PD-L1) treatment leads to clinical activity in metastatic bladder cancer. Nature 515(7528):558–562

26. Emens LA et al (2015) Abstract 2859: Inhibition of PD-L1 by MPDL3280A leads to clinical activity in patients with metastatic triple-negative breast cancer (TNBC). Cancer Res 75(15 suppl):2859

27. Hodi FS et al (2016) Evaluation of immune-related response criteria and RECIST v1.1 in patients with advanced melanoma treated with pembrolizumab. J Clin Oncol 34(13):1510–1517

28. Adams S et al (2016) Phase Ib trial of atezolizumab in combination with nab-paclitaxel in patients with metastatic triple-negative breast cancer (mTNBC). J Clin Oncol 34(15 suppl):1009

29. Emens LA et al (2016) IMpassion130: a Phase III randomized trial of atezolizumab with nab-paclitaxel for first-line treatment of patients with metastatic triple-negative breast cancer (mTNBC). J Clin Oncol 34(15 suppl): p. TPS1104-TPS1104

30. Dirix L et al (2016) Abstract S1-04: Avelumab (MSB0010718C), an anti-PD-L1 antibody, in patients with locally advanced or metastatic breast cancer: A phase Ib JAVELIN solid tumor trial. Cancer Res 76(4 suppl): p. S1-04-S1-04

Sexual Function Post-Breast Cancer

Lauren Streicher and James A. Simon

11

Contents

L. Streicher (✉) · J. A. Simon
The Northwestern Medicine Center for Sexual Medicine and Menopause,
Feinberg School of Medicine, Chicago, USA
e-mail: lstreicher@nm.org

J. A. Simon
George Washington University, Washington, USA

© Springer International Publishing AG 2018
W. J. Gradishar (ed.), *Optimizing Breast Cancer Management*, Cancer Treatment
and Research 173, https://doi.org/10.1007/978-3-319-70197-4_11

Abstract

The consequences of estrogen deprivation and therapeutic interventions such as radiation, chemotherapy and surgery have a significant negative impact on libido, sexual arousal, orgasmic function and the ability to have pleasurable intercourse. Evaluation and treatment of female sexual dysfunction is a significant unmet need in the breast cancer survivor in spite of the availability of safe and effective treatments.

Keywords

Female sexual dysfunction · Hypoactive sexual desire disorder · Dyspareunia Genitourinary syndrome of menopause · Vaginal estrogen · DHEA · Prasterone Ospemifene · Fractional CO2 laser

Up to seventy-five percent of breast cancer survivors report either transient or permanent physical, psychological or interpersonal sexual concerns [1]. Physical changes post-treatment effect body image along with the potential loss of erogenous sensations of the breast or genitals. Fatigue, insomnia, depression, and anxiety, as well as partner issues are contributing factors beyond physical and hormonal changes.

For many women, however, the consequences of iatrogenic menopause or estrogen deprivation therapy have the greatest negative impact on sexual function. Estrogen deprivation results in distressing vasomotor symptoms, sleep disturbance, and alterations in cognitive function that impact sexual desire and arousal. The effects of estrogen deprivation on genital tissue are profound and include, not only the loss of elasticity and lubrication required for pleasurable intercourse, but also impaired vascular function, which in turn impacts on arousal, and orgasmic function.

Sexual function is frequently relegated to a "low priority status" at the time of a breast cancer diagnosis and initial treatment. All too often however, sexual function remains a low priority once the patient is doing well even though this loss of sexual function is associated with significant distress, depression, and a negative impact on intimacy and personal relationships. It is important to keep in mind that forty percent of the general population report sexual problems and many cancer survivors struggled with sexual complaints long before their diagnosis and treatment [2]. While radiation, surgery, or chemotherapy may precipitate new onset sexual dysfunction, it often exacerbates an already existing problem.

While any cancer diagnosis and treatment can lead to high rates of sexual dysfunction from depression, chemotherapy and it's resultant fatigue, alopecia, hypoestrogenemia (either transient or permanent), and myelosuppression, and breast cancer is associated with additional unique sexual concerns as a result of body-altering breast surgery, endocrine therapy, and breast radiation.

11.1 Surgery

Body image and breast sensitivity are associated with both normal arousal, but also sexual desire, and the ability to achieve orgasm. Therefore, any breast altering surgery can negatively impact sexual function. In a prospective trial assessing the impact of breast-conserving therapy versus mastectomy [3], in comparison to healthy controls, no significant differences in sexual functioning were found after breast-conserving surgery. Significantly, more women who underwent mastectomy reported problems with sexual desire, arousal, the ability to achieve an orgasm, and the intensity of the orgasm. The impact of reconstructive surgery, including the timing of reconstructive surgery on sexual function is complex and multifactorial. One prospective study followed and compared the psychosexual function of 190 women who underwent mastectomy alone, mastectomy with immediate reconstruction, or mastectomy with delayed reconstruction [4]. Contrary to the assumed psychological benefits of breast reconstruction, psychological distress was evident among women regardless of reconstruction or timing of reconstruction. Sexual function was not different one-year post-surgery between women with mastectomy alone, mastectomy with immediate reconstruction, and delayed reconstruction.

The length of time post-surgery may be more important than the type or timing of reconstructive surgery. In another study of psychosocial parameters, including sexual function, six years after surgery, the differences between those with mastectomy alone and those who underwent postmastectomy delayed breast reconstruction showed improvement in both groups over the immediate post-op period [5].

Fat grafting as an adjunct to the breast reconstruction appears to be safe and may improve breast satisfaction and sexual well-being [6].

Risk-reducing bilateral oophorectomy, with or without hysterectomy, also has a profound effect on sexual function due to the onset of immediate and untreated menopausal symptoms. In addition, oophorectomy results in the loss of secreted ovarian androgens beyond what occurs in natural menopause [7].

Utilizing validated questionnaires in women with breast cancer who underwent risk-reducing surgery, 80% of women with breast cancer had sexual dysfunction, and 82% had hypoactive sexual desire disorder (HSDD). Many women in the study group also were using adjunctive endocrine therapies. Compared to tamoxifen, aromatase inhibitors were significantly associated with reduced lubrication, arousal, orgasm, and greater dyspareunia.

11.2 Radiation Therapy

It is often challenging to determine the effects of radiation therapy on sexual function since most women who undergo radiation treatment are also having breast surgery and/or chemotherapy. Nonetheless, the resultant chronic breast pain, alteration in breast skin and color, lymphedema, and shoulder pain from radiation therapy can impact body image and sexual functioning. A 2014 review of 633 women, 3 years post-radiation found that patients with radiation had significantly lowered sexual well-being compared with non-irradiated patients [8].

11.3 Endocrine Therapy

The treatment of women with hormone receptor-positive cancers often includes an aromatase inhibitor or selective estrogen receptor modulator, such as tamoxifen. These treatments can initiate or worsen menopausal symptoms such as vasomotor flashes, urinary symptoms, and vaginal atrophy. Dyspareunia and the inability to have penetrative vaginal intercourse are common sequelae [9]. The impact of tamoxifen therapy on sexual function varies widely, and its effect may be impacted by the ambient estrogenic and androgenic milieu at the time of initiation. Both estrogen and androgen production are highly variable and dependent upon the reproductive status of the pre, peri, and postmenopausal ovary. Up to 31% of tamoxifen-treated patients report dyspareunia.

Women taking aromatase inhibitors demonstrate significantly greater sexual dysfunction than women treated with tamoxifen. In a survey sent to women post-aromatase inhibitor therapy, ninety-three percent of women scored as dysfunctional on the Female Sexual Function Index (FSFI). About 75% of dysfunctional women were distressed about sexual problems [10]. Although only 52% of women were sexually active when starting their aromatase inhibitor, 79% of this group developed a new sexual problem including 24% who ceased to have part-nered sexual activity altogether.

In a population-based study of sexual function [9, 11], 4% of aromatase inhibitor-treated breast cancer patients were dissatisfied with their sex life in general, and 50.0% reported low sexual interest. 73.9% of aromatase inhibitor-treated patients reported insufficient lubrication. Dyspareunia was present in 56.5% of aromatase inhibitor-treated cases which was significantly more common than in controls, irrespective of hormonal use. Overall, the majority of women taking aromatase inhibitors have sexual dysfunction that is distressing and difficult to resolve.

Evaluation of sexual health in the breast cancer patient requires an understanding of the four categories of female sexual dysfunction.

11.4 Sexual Desire Disorders

Sexual desire disorders include both hypoactive sexual desire disorder (HSDD) and sexual aversion disorder. Hypoactive sexual desire disorder (HSDD) is defined as the persistent or recurrent deficiency or absence of sexual thoughts, fantasies, and/or desire for, or receptivity to, sexual activity which causes marked personal distress or interpersonal difficulties and is not better accounted for by another primary disorder, drug/medication, or general medical condition [12]. While this definition (from the DSM IV TR) is used here, HSDD was recently incorporated (with arousal disorder) into a unified disorder, female sexual interest, and arousal disorder (FSIAD) [12].

The cancer patient, strictly speaking, does not meet the criteria for HSDD since the lack of sexual desire can usually be explained by their chronic medical condition. Having said that, lack of libido or desire, regardless of etiology, is often distressing, and of great concern either because of a lost desire to desire sex (wanting to want) or the impact such a loss has on intimate relationships.

Diminished or absent libido in the cancer patient is typically multifactorial and is the result of any of the following:

Relationship problems
History of trauma or abuse
Medications, (particularly SSRIs and other psychotropic agents)
Depression
Sexual pain
Alcohol
Stress
Fatigue
Menopause
Co-morbidities such as hypothyroidism and incontinence.

11.5   Impaired Arousal

The current Diagnostic and Statistical Manual (DSM) includes the inability to become aroused as part of sexual desire disorder (see FSIAD, above). Many sexual health experts feel it is more appropriate to separate these categories since someone may have a strong libido (desires sexual activity), but does not experience the physical sensations of arousal. Arousal, a primarily vascular function, (vasodilation and increased blood flow) is easily reduced with loss of estrogen, and the subsequent impact estrogen deficiency has on the endothelial nitric oxide vasodilation pathway.

11.6   Orgasmic Disorder

Orgasmic disorder is defined as the persistence or recurrent delay in or absence of orgasm after normal excitement phase which causes marked distress or interpersonal difficulty [12]. While primary orgasmic disorder is included, most breast cancer survivors experience acquired hypo-orgasmia or anorgasmia.

The etiology of post-cancer orgasmic disorder may include any of the following:

SSRIs
Other medications (narcotics, benzodiazepines, lithium, etc.)
Dyspareunia
History of sexual trauma
Pelvic floor disorders
Menopause
Situational/Relationship
Medical co-morbidities (diabetic neuropathy, incontinence, vascular disease, hypothyroidism).

11.7   Sexual Pain Disorders

Sexual pain in the breast cancer patient includes superficial dyspareunia (pain upon insertion of a penis or "toy"), deep dyspareunia (deep pelvic pain with thrusting) or in many cases, both superficial and deep dyspareunia. Vaginismus (a largely discontinued term) is defined as a persistent difficulty to allow vaginal entry of a penis/finger/object, despite the woman's expressed wish to do so. Vaginismus is a result of variable involuntary pelvic floor muscle contraction in anticipation of or fear of pain.

Vaginismus is typically a secondary consequence of dyspareunia, or other prior sexual trauma, and it is essentially a protective mechanism (i.e., to "protect" one from anticipated pain). Even after the initial cause of the pain is treated and eliminated, vaginismus may be persistent, and require "re-education," using pelvic floor physical therapy to erase the "muscle memory."

While vulvovaginal atrophy from hypoestrogenemia is the most common cause of dyspareunia in the breast cancer patient, it is critical to identify all possible causes before assuming sexual pain is a result of atrophic vulvar or vaginal tissues.

11.8 Possible Causes of Superficial Dyspareunia

Estrogen deficiency (iatrogenic or natural)
Vulvovestibulodynias
Lichen sclerosus
Lichen planus
Female genital mutilation
Pelvic radiation
Chemotherapy Graft-versus-host reaction
Hypertonic pelvic floor
Vulvar dermatologic conditions
Vaginismus.

11.9 Possible Causes of Deep Dyspareunia

Endometriosis
Adhesions
Constipation
Irritable bowel syndrome
Ovarian cysts
Endometritis
Pelvic organ prolapse
Adenomyosis
Fibroids
Interstitial cystitis
Bladder cancer
Diverticular disease
Pelvic infections
Hypertonic pelvic floor.

11.10 History and Physical Examination

Studies consistently show that patients will rarely introduce the topic of sexual concerns, but patients are willing to discuss the topic once initiated by her physician or an advanced practice nurse [13]. Therefore, the onus is on the clinician to broach the topic. *Every patient*, whether they are partnered or single, and irrespective of sexual orientation, should be screened for sexual issues. Open-ended questions are often most effective in this regard. One approach is to simply state,

> Many women with cancer have sexual concerns…about their level of desire, pleasure during sexual activity or the ability to achieve orgasm. How are things going for you?

The **Better** Model was designed to aid in identifying cancer patients with sexual concerns [14].

B   *Bring up the topic*
E   *Explain that sexuality is part of quality of life and can be discussed*
T   *Tell patients resources will be provided*
T   *Timing, ask for information at any time*
E   *Educate about sexual side effects of Rx*
R   *Record.*

Alternatively, one might choose to use a sexual health screener. While the 19 question Female Sexual Function Index (FSFI-questionaire.com) [15] is typically utilized in sexual health practices, and for research, a much shorter validated version is usually adequate to identify which patients have such problems and desire treatment.

Sexual Symptom Checklist for Women

Please answer the following questions about your overall sexual function:

1. Are you satisfied with your sexual function?   ❑ Yes   ❑ No

If no, please continue.

2. How long have you been dissatisfied with your sexual function? _____

3. Mark which of the following problems you are having, and circle the one that is most bothersome:
   ❑ Little or no interest in sex
   ❑ Decreased genital sensation (feeling)
   ❑ Decreased vaginal lubrication (dryness)
   ❑ Problem reaching orgasm
   ❑ Pain during sex
   ❑ Other: _____

4. Would you like to talk about it with your doctor?   ❑ Yes   ❑ No

---

In addition, a psychological evaluation by a therapist who is trained in, not only the psychological ramifications, but also the physical, hormonal, and medical ramifications of breast cancer treatment, ideally should be a part of the evaluation. The American Association of Sexuality Educators, Counselors and Therapists (ASSECT) certify licensed mental health professionals who have been trained to provide in-depth psychotherapy and who specialize in treating patients with sexual issues and concerns.

ASSECT-certified therapists utilize these four steps. The P-LI-SS-IT Model is as follows:

Permission (P): The practitioner creates a climate of comfort and permission for clients to discuss sexual concerns, often introducing the topic of sexuality, thereby validating sexuality as a legitimate health issue.
Limited information (LI): The practitioner addresses specific sexual concerns and attempts to correct myths and misinformation.
Specific suggestions (SS): The practitioner compiles a sexual history or profile of the client.

The therapist can then assist the client in formulating perceptions and ideas about sources of these concerns and collaborate with healthcare providers to develop realistic and appropriate goals and solution plans.

11.11 Physical Examination

A targeted systematic physical examination of the female cancer patient with sexual concerns is an essential and early component of an effective treatment plan. Evaluation without physical examination can result in misdiagnosis and failed treatment of sexual function problems. A 2016 review in the journal CA: includes a detailed description of the physical examination of the patient with sexual concerns [16]. This comprehensive physical examination is ideally performed by a practitioner other than the breast surgeon and should include a detailed survey of the vulva, clitoris, vaginal mucosa, vaginal pH, vaginal walls, pelvic floor, and pelvic organs.

11.12 Treatment

Not everyone with sexual dysfunction wants treatment. The decision to proceed is often a balance between perceived need ("How important is this really") and concern about the treatment. ("The last thing I need right now is more invasive treatments or medication that may have dangerous or undesirable side effects.") If a patient declines treatment, give her resources and let her know that she may choose to explore options at another time. The medical, surgical, and radiation oncologist are typically the primary medical point of contact but often are not equipped to manage the myriad of sexual issues that are consequences of breast cancer treatment. Collaboration with a certified sex therapist addresses the psychosocial and relationship issues that inevitably occur from the hormonal, medical, and physical impact of breast cancer and breast cancer therapy. If a patient chooses to proceed with treatment, a referral to a gynecologist or sexual health expert is appropriate.

However, oncologists should still be familiar with pharmacologic therapies even if they do not prescribe them since the patient will generally ask for her oncologist's approval if another specialist makes a recommendation.

11.13   Treatment of Sexual Pain

Superficial dyspareunia is the most common type of pain experienced during intercourse and is generally the consequence of atrophic vulvar and vaginal tissues from hypoestrogenemia and/or chemotherapy. In 2013, the terminology *vulvovaginal atrophy* was replaced by the term *genitourinary syndrome of menopause* which includes a description of symptoms in addition to anatomic changes and also acknowledges that postmenopause urinary symptoms such as frequency, burning, urgency, and recurrent urinary tract infections are a consequence of hypoestrogenemia [17].

Genitourinary Syndrome of Menopause

SYMPTOMS

- Genital dryness
- Decreased lubrication with IC
- Discomfort with Sexual Activity
- Irritation, burning, Itching
- Dysuria
- Urinary frequency, urgency
- Recurrent UTI

SIGNS

- Decreased moisture
- Decreased elasticity
- Labial resorption
- Pallor/Erythema
- Loss of vaginal rugae
- Mucosal fragility, petechiae
- pH >5
- Maturation Index:
  - Decreased superficial layer, increased parabasal layer

11.14   Lubricants

Lubricants are generally the first option to alleviate sexual pain due to vaginal dryness and difficult vaginal penetration. Lubricants and vaginal moisturizers are often lumped together, even though they are intended to serve very different purposes.

A lubricant is to be used at the time of intercourse to reduce friction. Lubricants work immediately and are not absorbed and are generally applied to the introitus and to the penis as opposed to being placed directly inside the vaginal canal. A long-acting vaginal moisturizer, on the other hand, is applied inside the vagina, on a regular basis, in anticipation of intercourse and is intended to change the properties of the vaginal mucosa as opposed to simply providing a slippery barrier.

Many lubricants call themselves moisturizers as a marketing strategy since women may be more comfortable buying a moisturizer than a lubricant. The only way to know what the product is and what it is intended to do is to read the ingredients and the description of where it is to be applied. Many women, prior to consulting a clinician, have already tried "home products" such as petroleum jelly, cooking oils, or baby oil. While fine for occasional use, these products may increase the risk of candidiasis and bacterial vaginosis [18]. In addition, oil-based or petroleum products are not latex condom compatible. Patients should be advised to only use products that are intended for vaginal use.

The basic categories of commercially available lubricants include water-based, silicone-based, hyaluronic acid-based, and oil-based. Hybrid lubricants combine water and silicone. Silicone and water-based lubricants are typically condom compatible. Oil-based lubricants are not.

11.15 Water-Based Lubricants

Water-based lubricants are inexpensive and readily available. For many women, they are adequate; however, since they tend to become sticky, as the water dries out, and require multiple applications, water-based lubricants are often insufficient.

Most water-based lubricants contain glycerin. While it is often stated that glycerin promotes vaginal yeast infections, there is no data to support that concern [19]. Propylene glycol is a preservative commonly added to lubricants of all kinds, particularly water-based varieties, which some women find irritating and should be avoided, particularly in women post-chemotherapy.

Pre-Seed® is a water-based lubricant intended for women trying to conceive since it does not inhibit sperm mobility. It is often the preferred lubricant of women post-chemotherapy since this iso-osmotic product is preservative-free.

11.16 Silicone-Based Lubricants

Silicone lubricants are generally preferred since they are very slippery, long-lasting, and generally non-irritating. A minor negative is that silicone lubricants cannot be used with silicone covered or formed vaginal toys or devices, since they will react with and breakdown the silicone. Some women will put a condom over the toy to protect it.

11.17 "Specialty" Lubricants

Flavored lubricants, warming lubricants, and stimulating lubricants can be highly irritating and generally should be avoided.

The following examples of products are available over the counter are non-irritating and condom compatible.

11.18 Water-Based Lubricants

PINK water
Liquid silk
YES water-based
Sliquid organics natural
Astroglide
JO water-based
PJUR water-based
Pre-Seed.

Silicone Lubricants

Replens silky smooth
Wet platinum
JO premium personal lubricant
PINK silicone lubricant
SLIQUID organics silk
PJUR eros woman bodyglide
Swiss navy silicone.

11.19 Moisturizers

A true long-acting vaginal moisturizer is intended to alter vaginal mucosa by increasing intracellular water content, and provide elasticity, and lubrication. In spite of claims from dozens of products that call themselves "moisturizers," most products labeled as "personal," or "feminine" moisturizers are actually vulvar, as opposed to vaginal moisturizers or lubricants. Only one product, Replens, intended for vaginal, not vulvar use, has been shown in clinical trials to increase vaginal elasticity and lubrication [20]. Replens contains polycarbophil, a bio-adhesive that adheres to vaginal mucosa and promotes intracellular water absorption. Polycarbophil is also a weak acid that buffers vaginal tissues to lower the vaginal pH to between 3 and 4.5 allowing repopulation with lactobacilli. Replens is the only long-acting moisturizer that has been approved by the FDA, and like local vaginal estrogens has been shown to lower pH and decrease dyspareunia. Many women who are not sexually active use Replens to reduce chronic vaginal irritation and infections which can result in urinary tract infections as well.

Hyaluronic acid vaginal gel is another over the counter long-acting moisturizer that is used to alleviate vaginal dryness. In a small open-label trial, hyaluronic acid worked as well as estriol (but not as well as topical estradiol) to relieve vaginal itching, burning, and dyspareunia [21].

While lubricants and moisturizers are adequate for women with mild atrophy, severe atrophy generally requires a pharmacologic intervention to repair the tissue.

11.20 Low-Dose Vaginal Estrogen

Due to the current class labeling of all estrogen pharmaceutical products, one would be led to believe that low-dose vaginal estrogen products are contraindicated for women with a history of breast cancer [22]. These erroneous risk profiles associated with higher systemic doses are not consistent with local treatments that minimize the risk of systemic estrogen absorption [23].

Systemic absorption is dependent on the degree of vaginal atrophy and the pharmaceutical formulation used [24]. The degree of vaginal atrophy is dependent on the fragility of the vaginal epithelium and the loss of superficial cells. Estrogen absorption decreases as the integrity of the vaginal epithelium improves and the tissue thickens [23]. For local dosing, a little goes a long way and continued, regular use of a low-dose vaginal estrogen is effective to sustain the positive tissue effects with minimal systemic absorption [25]. Low-dose vaginal estrogen is available as vaginal tablets, rings, and creams. Vaginal tablets or rings produce the lowest rate of systemic absorption. Additionally, they have the benefit of a set dosing regimen that eliminates user over-application that may occur with creams. Creams offer the option for variable dosing, which can be particularly useful for a patient with severe hypoestrogenic atrophy effecting the vulvar tissue and requiring spot application. Although there is an increased systemic absorption with cream use, no increase in breast cancer recurrence has been associated regardless of dose used [26].

In 2016, The American College of Obstetricians and Gynecologists (ACOG) issued a committee opinion regarding use of low-dose vaginal estrogens in woman experiencing genitourinary symptoms with a history of estrogen-dependent breast cancer and those undergoing breast cancer treatments [27]. It states that in the event that urogenital symptoms cannot be relieved with non-hormonal approaches that low-dose vaginal estrogens in a ring or tablet preparation could be appropriate when used in consultation with the patient's oncologist. The currently available data, including a large scale, nested-case, controlled cohort study of breast cancer survivors receiving a variety of endocrine treatments [28], does not support any increased risk of cancer recurrence for women utilizing vaginal estrogen [29]. The safety threshold for systemic estrogen levels for survivors of breast cancer is still unknown [30], but the change in serum estrogen levels associated with vaginal tablets and rings in women taking aromatase inhibitors and tamoxifen is both minimal and transient [29, 31].

11.21 Ospemifene

Ospemifene is a relatively new pharmaceutical option for the treatment of moderate to severe dyspareunia due to estrogen deficiency. As a selective estrogen receptor modulator (SERM), it is well suited for the treatment of dyspareunia in women with a history of breast cancer because of its estrogen-like agonistic effects on the vulvar and vaginal tissue, weak action, if any, on the endometrium without clinical significance, and an antagonistic (antiestrogenic) effects on breast tissue [32, 33]. Although there is limited data on the long-term effects of ospemifene and only a small number of women with a history of breast cancer were included in the clinical trials, no clinically significant changes in breast outcomes and no recurrence of breast cancer have been reported [34–38]. While ospemifene is contraindicated for use during estrogen-dependent cancer treatment, it can be used safely after adjuvant treatment has been successfully completed [33].

11.22 Vaginal DHEA

The most novel, and recently FDA-approved vaginal atrophy treatment is vaginal prasterone, also known as dehydroepiandrosterone (DHEA) [39, 40]. In postmenopausal women, DHEA is a systemically inactive precursor to all sex hormones [41]. Since DHEA undergoes intracrinological processes at target tissues, vaginal DHEA results in active sex steroids exclusively within the vaginal tissue without systemic involvement [42]. This targeted response would make DHEA a highly desirable treatment for atrophy in patients with a current or past history of breast cancer. While it has been confirmed that the FDA-approved dose of DHEA does, in fact, limit the systemic exposure to elevated serum sex hormone concentrations, additional study would be required to fully elucidate the safety profile of vaginal DHEA in breast cancer patients and survivors [11, 43].

11.23 Fractional CO_2 Laser Treatments

The CO_2 laser has been available for years as a method to reduce facial wrinkles, remove tattoos, and treat a myriad of skin conditions. In 2014, the CO_2 laser became FDA cleared for "incision, excision, ablation, vaporization, and coagulation of body soft tissues in medical specialties including… aesthetic (dermatology and plastic surgery), gynecology…"

The mechanism of action is similar in all tissues treated with the CO_2 laser. Fractionated beams of light penetrate small areas of tissue to create small ablative wounds in the epithelium and underlying lamina propria. There is sufficient energy so lateral "spared tissue" is also treated. The depth of the laser energy is modulated so that the treatment is confined to the mucosa and lamina propria. Wounding the tissue stimulates collagen remodeling and regeneration. Repair mechanisms such as chemotaxis, neo-collagenesis, angiogenesis, epithelialization, and glycosamino-glycans (GAG) formation are then activated. Histologic examination and gross examination of post-treatment vaginal mucosa are indistinguishable from estroge-nized tissue with restoration of superficial epithelium, rugae, and lubrication [44].

Treatment of both vaginal and vulvar tissues is performed without anesthesia in an office setting and takes approximately five minutes. A 10 cm tube-shaped vaginal probe is placed in the vagina, rotated and withdrawn at 1 cm intervals, in order to treat the entire vaginal canal. An external probe is then used to treat the vestibule and vulva as needed. The protocol includes three treatments spaced at 6-week intervals. A careful pre- and post-treatment evaluation is essential since all sexual pain is not secondary to tissue atrophy.

Despite a paucity of data, the CO_2 laser has been increasingly available as an appropriate option for the treatment of sexual pain due to vulvar vaginal atrophy. The first US trial measured Vaginal Wall Elasticity (Dilator Evaluation), FSFI, QOL, and PGI Patient Global Impression of Improvement [45]. About 96% of women were reportedly satisfied or extremely satisfied at follow-up, and 83% showed increase in comfortable dilator size at three-month follow-up. Dryness and dyspareunia showed the most improvement, with statistically significant improve-ment in vaginal health index scores and the validated Female Sexual Function Index (FSFI). Findings were consistent with those previously demonstrated in earlier European studies [46].

In addition to treating dryness and dyspareunia, emerging data also shows benefit in urinary symptoms such as urgency, burning, and recurrent urinary tract infections. There is also preliminary evidence that the CO_2 laser is useful in the treatment of recurrent vaginitis and lichen sclerosis. No significant safety issues or adverse reactions have been reported. It is uncertain how long the effects of the treatment will last. The companies that distribute the lasers recommend an annual "booster" treatment, but there is no data to support this. A twelve-month follow-up did show persistence of treatment effect [47].

While more data and sham-controlled studies are needed, the CO_2 laser is a promising option for women who have been advised, or prefer, not to use a sys-temic vaginal selective estrogen receptor modulator, prasterone, or a local vaginal estrogen product. The CO_2 laser is a medical, not a cosmetic device, and should not be used for vaginal "rejuvenation" or "tightening," The CO_2 laser is also not indicated for the treatment of stress incontinence, sexual satisfaction in the absence of atrophy, low libido, impaired arousal, or orgasmic dysfunction.

As with any other treatment, post-laser evaluation is essential since all sexual pain is not secondary to tissue atrophy. Persistent pain post-treatment requires a thorough investigation to rule out other causes of dyspareunia including high-tone pelvic floor dysfunction and/or vaginismus secondary to years of sexual pain. Modalities such as pelvic floor physical therapy and dilator therapy are often required. Sex therapy is also a useful adjunct.

Given the significant unmet need, fractional CO_2 laser therapy is an appropriate option for many patients.

11.24 Pelvic Floor PT

Once vaginal and vulvar tissues have regained elasticity and lubrication, pelvic floor physical therapy is commonly required to treat pelvic floor dysfunction that develops as a result of painful intercourse. The pelvic floor muscles contract inappropriately as a defense mechanism, and eliminating the muscle memory is needed to eliminate dyspareunia. In addition, dilator therapy is often required to regain tissue elasticity and eliminate vaginismus.

The experienced pelvic physical therapist not only treats the problem but also plays an important role in determining the source of pain. In performing a thorough musculoskeletal evaluation of the pelvis, spine, and hips, she often finds pelvic asymmetry and muscle imbalances in women with pelvic and sexual pain. Often the location of the pain is not where the pelvic pain originates. For example, tight hip flexor muscles tilt the pelvis and cause tension in the pelvic floor muscles, which contribute, in turn, to pelvic pain and dysfunction.

Once the source of the pain is identified, the therapist uses a number of modalities for treatment, including techniques such as biofeedback, electrical stimulation, myofascial release, and joint mobilization. Muscle spasms are eliminated using manual soft tissue work, and trigger point release directly on the pelvic floor muscles through the vagina or rectum. These techniques really work to eliminate pain, improve tissue integrity via increased circulation and tissue oxygenation, and restore normal resting muscle tone, and length.

If your institution does not have pelvic floor physical therapists, one can be located by going to www.hermanwallace.com, or to the American Physical Therapy Association website, www.womenshealthapta.org.

11.25 Treatment of Low Sexual Desire

The treatment for low sexual desire needs to be personalized to the each patient's needs, which will be dependent on their psychological state, current and past pathology and therapies, and relationship status. For patients with a current or past history of breast cancer or undergoing adjuvant treatment, the presentation of low sexual desire can be complex and may require the empiric use of multiple therapies prior to resolution. As discussed above, cancer patients and survivors do not strictly meet the definition for HSDD, but the course of treatment and common therapeutic options for HSDD may be appropriate for addressing their low desire.

11.26 Sex Therapy and Counseling

For all instances of low sexual desire without a sexual pain etiology, the first line of therapy is education and counseling. Identifying areas of intervention with the help of a trained sex or couples therapist to expand a patient's personal sexual knowledge, to explore areas that are hindering a patient's sexual desire, and to work with the patient's partner in understanding the issue of low sexual desire. Elucidating what will likely be a multifactorial cause of low desire in a current cancer patient or cancer survivor will determine the next therapeutics steps. While not well-supported by randomized controlled trials, cognitive therapy (e.g., cognitive behavior therapy, motivational interviewing, mindfulness training) alone has been shown to improve sexual desire outcomes, but the efficacy of these methods should be revisited in a more stringent manner [48].

11.27 Anti-depressants

Some anti-depressants exhibit properties which may be of interest for the treatment of low sexual desire such as increasing the response to sexual cues (e.g. bupropion, other dopamine agonists) or reducing the inhibitory response to sexual cues (e.g. trazodone, buspirone). A number of randomized controlled trials to explore the benefit of such off-label are used to improve sexual desire in both depressed and non-depressed populations of women [49]. For the breast cancer patient and survivor population, specifically, depression may already be a serious concern and the prescribed anti-depressant (e.g., selective serotonin and norepinephrine reuptake inhibitors, selective serotonin reuptake inhibitors) may be a contributing factor to decreased libido. Working with a patient's psychiatrist to adjust these medications toward a libido/sexual desire-friendly anti-depressant may improve or solve her low desire.

11.28 Testosterone

Use of testosterone for the treatment of low desire in women has been studied in great detail and off-label prescriptions in the USA is increasing [50, 51]. The 2014 Endocrine Society clinical practice guidelines express a favorable opinion for the use of testosterone for postmenopausal women with female sexual dysfunction with extensive evidence that testosterone therapy influences all aspects of sexual response [52]. This was a change from a prior recommendation that was influenced by the additional positive results from clinical studies of a transdermal testosterone patch demonstrating both safety and efficacy. Randomized, double-blind, placebo-controlled trials of transdermal testosterone patches (300 μg/day) for use in surgically [53–56], and naturally [57] menopausal women with HSDD with and without systemic estrogen hormone therapy [58] have shown increases in satisfying sexual events, increases in sexual desire, and decreases in personal distress with minimal adverse consequences.

To date, neither transdermal nor other testosterone studies have been conducted in women with a history of breast cancer. In women taking aromatase inhibitors, vaginal testosterone has been explored as an alternative to estrogen [59]. Dahir and Travers-Gustafson [60] showed statistically significant increases in all sexual domains using the FSFI as the patient reported outcome. A study utilizing the same dosing regimen in a similar population observed no appreciable change in serum estradiol levels with the majority of the levels undetectable by assay [61]. For women with a current or prior history of breast cancer, the safety of testosterone use is not fully understood, and additional study is required to determine testosterone's effect on the breast [52, 59]. For women who wish to pursue testosterone therapy, full disclosure of the unknown risks is necessary.

11.29 Flibanserin

The proposed etiology of HSDD is a dysfunction of the normal excitatory or inhibitory processes in the central nervous system (CNS) [62]. Arnow et al. [63] visualized this abnormal neuromodulation in women with HSDD using functional magnetic resonance imaging (fMRI) to show that women with HSDD showed increased activation in the medial frontal gyrus and the right inferior gyrus when presented with erotic stimuli compared to controls with no history of HSDD. These results suggest an overall "overthinking" to erotic stimuli with increased response inhibition and increased attention response.

In 2015, flibanserin became the first FDA-approved medication for the treatment HSDD in premenopausal women. Flibanserin is non-hormonal, postsynaptic serotonin 1A agonist/2A antagonist that acts in a localized fashion to decrease serotonin, and increase dopamine, and norepinephrine in the prefrontal cortex [64]. As a non-hormonal option, flibanserin would be a reasonable option for the breast cancer survivor. It has been demonstrated to significantly increase the frequency of satisfying sexual events, increase sexual desire, and reduce sexually related personal distress. Regardless of the FDA approval, limited to premenopausal women, there has been substantial positive data from a large-scale randomized controlled trials to suggest that use in postmenopausal women would be safe and efficacious [65]. Also, trial participants experienced few mild-to-moderate adverse events, including dizziness, somnolence, nausea, and headache, similar to the premenopausal trial participants [66–68].

Due in part to the perceived risk of hypotension and syncope with alcohol consumption, the FDA has implemented mandatory Risk Evaluation and Mitigation Strategies (REMS) for flibanserin prescribers [69]. Ultimately, this program limits the providers that are able to prescribe flibanserin, and therefore a patient who may benefit from flibanserin use may require a referral to a certified provider for therapeutic management. Response to flibanserin can be assessed after an 8-week treatment course at which point the decision to continue treatment should be made in consultation with the certified provider.

11.30 Future Options

For physicians who consult with patients with female sexual dysfunction, off-label treatments are common. The approval of flibanserin was revolutionary for both practitioners and patients alike. Hopefully, flibanserin will be joined by additional FDA-approved therapeutic options in the future. One such treatment is bremelanotide, an as-needed peptide melanocortin receptor agonist that modulates sexual CNS pathways for response [70]. It has been shown to elicit significant arousal responses in premenopausal [71, 72] and postmenopausal women [73]. With a minimal adverse event profile of nausea, flushing, headache, and injection site pain [72] and no hormonal interactions. Bremelanotide may be an ideal solution to female sexual dysfunction for women experiencing a situational decrease in sexual desire and/or arousal associated with breast cancer diagnosis and treatment. Palatin Technologies Inc. has announced plans to submit a New Drug Application to the FDA by the end of 2017 [74].

References

1. Raggio GA, Butryn ML, Arigo D, Mikorski R, Palmer SC (2014) Prevalence and correlates of sexual morbidity in long-term breast cancer survivors. Psychol Health 29:632–650
2. Shifren JL, Monz BU, Russo PA, Segreti A, Johannes CB (2008) Sexual problems and distress in United States women: prevalence and correlates. Obstet Gynecol 112:970–978
3. Aerts L, Christiaens MR, Enzlin P, Neven P, Amant F (2014) Sexual functioning in women after mastectomy versus breast conserving therapy for early-stage breast cancer: a prospective controlled study. Breast 23:629–636
4. Metcalfe KA, Semple J, Quan ML, Vadaparampil ST, Holloway C, Brown M et al (2012) Changes in psychosocial functioning 1 year after mastectomy alone, delayed breast reconstruction, or immediate breast reconstruction. Ann Surg Oncol 19:233–241
5. Metcalfe KA, Zhong T, Narod SA, Quan ML, Holloway C, Hofer S et al (2015) A prospective study of mastectomy patients with and without delayed breast reconstruction: long-term psychosocial functioning in the breast cancer survivorship period. J Surg Oncol 111:258–264
6. Bennet K, Qi J, Kim H (2017) Association of fat grafting with patient-reported outcomes in post mastectomy breast reconstruction. JAMA Surg. doi:10.1001/jamasurg.2017.1716
7. Tucker PE, Saunders C, Bulsara MK, Tan JJ, Salfinger SG, Green H et al (2016) Sexuality and quality of life in women with a prior diagnosis of breast cancer after risk-reducing salpingo-oophorectomy. Breast 30:26–31
8. Albornoz CR, Matros E, McCarthy CM, Klassen A, Cano SJ, Alderman AK et al (2014) Implant breast reconstruction and radiation: a multicenter analysis of long-term health-related quality of life and satisfaction. Ann Surg Oncol 21:2159–2164
9. Baumgart J, Nilsson K, Evers AS, Kallak TK, Poromaa IS (2013) Sexual dysfunction in women on adjuvant endocrine therapy after breast cancer. Menopause 20:162–168

10. Schover LR, Baum GP, Fuson LA, Brewster A, Melhem-Bertrandt A (2014) Sexual problems during the first 2 years of adjuvant treatment with aromatase inhibitors. J Sex Med 11: 3102–3111

11. Labrie F, Martel C (2017) A low dose (6.5 mg) of intravaginal DHEA permits a strictly local action while maintaining all serum estrogens or androgens as well as their metabolites within normal values. Horm Mol Biol Clin Investig 01(29):39–60

12. Diagnostic and Statistical Manual of Mental Disorders, 5th ed. American Psychiatric Association, Arlington, VA (2013)

13. Bachmann GA, Leiblum SR, Grill J (1989) Brief sexual inquiry in gynecologic practice. Obstet Gynecol 73:425–427

14. Katz A (2005) The sounds of silence: sexuality information for cancer patients. J Clin Oncol 23:238–241

15. Rosen R, Brown C, Heiman J, Leiblum S, Meston C, Shabsigh R et al (2000) The Female Sexual Function Index (FSFI): a multidimensional self-report instrument for the assessment of female sexual function. J Sex Marital Ther 26:191–208

16. Lindau ST, Abramsohn EM, Baron SR, Florendo J, Haefner HK, Jhingran A et al (2016) Physical examination of the female cancer patient with sexual concerns: what oncologists and patients should expect from consultation with a specialist. CA Cancer J Clin 66:241–263

17. Portman DJ, Gass ML (2014) Genitourinary syndrome of menopause: new terminology for vulvovaginal atrophy from the International Society for the Study of Women's Sexual Health and the North American Menopause Society. Maturitas 79:349–354

18. Brown JM, Hess KL, Brown S, Murphy C, Waldman AL, Hezareh M (2013) Intravaginal practices and risk of bacterial vaginosis and candidiasis infection among a cohort of women in the United States. Obstet Gynecol 121:773–780

19. Strandberg KL, Peterson ML, Lin YC, Pack MC, Chase DJ, Schlievert PM (2010) Glycerol monolaurate inhibits Candida and Gardnerella vaginalis in vitro and in vivo but not Lactobacillus. Antimicrob Agents Chemother 54:597–601

20. van der Laak JA, de Bie LM, de Leeuw H, de Wilde PC, Hanselaar AG (2002) The effect of Replens on vaginal cytology in the treatment of postmenopausal atrophy: cytomorphology versus computerised cytometry. J Clin Pathol 55:446–451

21. Chen J, Geng L, Song X, Li H, Giordan N, Liao Q (2013) Evaluation of the efficacy and safety of hyaluronic acid vaginal gel to ease vaginal dryness: a multicenter, randomized, controlled, open-label, parallel-group, clinical trial. J Sex Med 10:1575–1584

22. Manson JE, Goldstein SR, Kagan R, Kaunitz AM, Liu JH, Pinkerton JV et al (2014) Why the product labeling for low-dose vaginal estrogen should be changed. Menopause 21:911–916

23. Santen RJ (2015) Vaginal administration of estradiol: effects of dose, preparation and timing on plasma estradiol levels. Climacteric 18:121–134

24. Palacios S, Castelo-Branco C, Currie H, Mijatovic V, Nappi RE, Simon J et al (2015) Update on management of genitourinary syndrome of menopause: a practical guide. Maturitas 82:308–313

25. Sturdee DW, Panay N (2010) Recommendations for the management of postmenopausal vaginal atrophy. Climacteric 13:509–522

26. O'Meara ES, Rossing MA, Daling JR, Elmore JG, Barlow WE, Weiss NS (2001) Hormone replacement therapy after a diagnosis of breast cancer in relation to recurrence and mortality. J Natl Cancer Inst 93:754–762

27. ACOG Committee Opinion: Number 659 (2016) The use of vaginal estrogen in women with a history of estrogen-dependent breast cancer. Obstet Gynecol 127:e93–e96

28. Le Ray I, Dell'Aniello S, Bonnetain F, Azoulay L, Suissa S (2012) Local estrogen therapy and risk of breast cancer recurrence among hormone-treated patients: a nested case-control study. Breast Cancer Res Treat 135:603–609

29. Ponzone R, Biglia N, Jacomuzzi ME, Maggiorotto F, Mariani L, Sismondi P (2005) Vaginal oestrogen therapy after breast cancer: is it safe? Eur J Cancer 41:2673–2681

30. Trinkaus M, Chin S, Wolfman W, Simmons C, Clemons M (2008) Should urogenital atrophy in breast cancer survivors be treated with topical estrogens? Oncologist 13:222–231
31. Wills S, Ravipati A, Venuturumilli P, Kresge C, Folkerd E, Dowsett M et al (2012) Effects of vaginal estrogens on serum estradiol levels in postmenopausal breast cancer survivors and women at risk of breast cancer taking an aromatase inhibitor or a selective estrogen receptor modulator. J Oncol Pract 8:144–148
32. Gennari L, Merlotti D, Valleggi F, Nuti R (2009) Ospemifene use in postmenopausal women. Expert Opin Investig Drugs 18:839–849
33. Nappi RE, Murina F, Perrone G, Villa P, Biglia N (2017) Clinical profile of women with vulvar and vaginal atrophy who are not candidates for local vaginal estrogen therapy. Minerva Ginecol 69:370–380
34. Simon J, Portman D, Mabey RG Jr (2014) Long-term safety of ospemifene (52-week extension) in the treatment of vulvar and vaginal atrophy in hysterectomized postmenopausal women. Maturitas 77:274–281
35. Simon JA, Lin VH, Radovich C, Bachmann GA (2013) One-year long-term safety extension study of ospemifene for the treatment of vulvar and vaginal atrophy in postmenopausal women with a uterus. Menopause 20:418–427
36. Portman D, Palacios S, Nappi RE, Mueck AO (2014) Ospemifene, a non-oestrogen selective oestrogen receptor modulator for the treatment of vaginal dryness associated with postmenopausal vulvar and vaginal atrophy: a randomised, placebo-controlled, phase III trial. Maturitas 78:91–98
37. Goldstein SR, Bachmann GA, Koninckx PR, Lin VH, Portman DJ, Ylikorkala O (2014) Ospemifene 12-month safety and efficacy in postmenopausal women with vulvar and vaginal atrophy. Climacteric 17:173–182
38. Berga SL (2013) Profile of ospemifene in the breast. Reprod Sci 20:1130–1136
39. Labrie F, Archer DF, Koltun W, Vachon A, Young D, Frenette L et al (2016) Efficacy of intravaginal dehydroepiandrosterone (DHEA) on moderate to severe dyspareunia and vaginal dryness, symptoms of vulvovaginal atrophy, and of the genitourinary syndrome of menopause. Menopause 23:243–256
40. Kaufman MB (2017) Pharmaceutical approval update. P T 42:90–91
41. Labrie F, Martel C, Balser J (2011) Wide distribution of the serum dehydroepiandrosterone and sex steroid levels in postmenopausal women: role of the ovary? Menopause 18:30–43
42. Martel C, Labrie F, Archer DF, Ke Y, Gonthier R, Simard JN et al (2016) Serum steroid concentrations remain within normal postmenopausal values in women receiving daily 6.5 mg intravaginal prasterone for 12weeks. J Steroid Biochem Mol Biol 159:142–153
43. Lester J, Pahouja G, Andersen B, Lustberg M (2015) Atrophic vaginitis in breast cancer survivors: a difficult survivorship issue. J Personalized Med 5:50–66
44. Zerbinati N, Serati M, Origoni M, Candiani M, Iannitti T, Salvatore S et al (2015) Microscopic and ultrastructural modifications of postmenopausal atrophic vaginal mucosa after fractional carbon dioxide laser treatment. Lasers Med Sci 30:429–436
45. Sokol ER, Karram MM (2016) An assessment of the safety and efficacy of a fractional CO2 laser system for the treatment of vulvovaginal atrophy. Menopause 23:1102–1107
46. Salvatore S, Nappi RE, Parma M, Chionna R, Lagona F, Zerbinati N et al (2015) Sexual function after fractional microablative CO(2) laser in women with vulvovaginal atrophy. Climacteric 18:219–225
47. Sokol ER, Karram MM (2016) Use of a novel fractional CO_2 laser for the treatment of genitourinary syndrome of menopause: 1-year outcomes. Menopause 24:810–814
48. Pyke RE, Clayton AH (2015) Psychological treatment trials for hypoactive sexual desire disorder: a sexual medicine critique and perspective. J Sex Med 12:2451–2458
49. Kingsberg SA, Clayton AH, Pfaus JG (2015) The female sexual response: current models, neurobiological underpinnings and agents currently approved or under investigation for the treatment of hypoactive sexual desire disorder. CNS Drugs 29:915–933

50. Snabes MC, Simes SM (2009) Approved hormonal treatments for HSDD: an unmet medical need. J Sex Med 6:1846–1849
51. Khera M (2015) Testosterone therapy for female sexual dysfunction. Sex Med Rev 3:137–144
52. Wierman ME, Arlt W, Basson R, Davis SR, Miller KK, Murad MH et al (2014) Androgen therapy in women: a reappraisal: an Endocrine Society clinical practice guideline. J Clin Endocrinol Metab 99:3489–3510
53. Buster JE, Kingsberg SA, Aguirre O, Brown C, Breaux JG, Buch A et al (2005) Testosterone patch for low sexual desire in surgically menopausal women: a randomized trial. Obstet Gynecol 105:944–952
54. Kingsberg S (2007) Testosterone treatment for hypoactive sexual desire disorder in postmenopausal women. J Sex Med 4(Suppl 3):227–234
55. Braunstein GD, Sundwall DA, Katz M, Shifren JL, Buster JE, Simon JA et al (2005) Safety and efficacy of a testosterone patch for the treatment of hypoactive sexual desire disorder in surgically menopausal women: a randomized, placebo-controlled trial. Arch Intern Med 165:1582–1589
56. Simon J, Braunstein G, Nachtigall L, Utian W, Katz M, Miller S et al (2005) Testosterone patch increases sexual activity and desire in surgically menopausal women with hypoactive sexual desire disorder. J Clin Endocrinol Metab 90:5226–5233
57. Shifren JL, Davis SR, Moreau M, Waldbaum A, Bouchard C, DeRogatis L et al (2006) Testosterone patch for the treatment of hypoactive sexual desire disorder in naturally menopausal women: results from the INTIMATE NM1 Study. Menopause 13:770–779
58. Davis SR, Moreau M, Kroll R, Bouchard C, Panay N, Gass M et al (2008) Testosterone for low libido in postmenopausal women not taking estrogen. N Engl J Med 359:2005–2017
59. Lemke EA, Madsen LT, Dains JE (2017) Vaginal testosterone for management of aromatase inhibitor-related sexual dysfunction: an integrative review. Oncol Nurs Forum 44:296–301
60. Dahir M, Travers-Gustafson D (2014) Breast cancer, aromatase inhibitor therapy, and sexual functioning: a pilot study of the effects of vaginal testosterone therapy. Sex Med 2:8–15
61. Witherby S, Johnson J, Demers L, Mount S, Littenberg B, Maclean CD et al (2011) Topical testosterone for breast cancer patients with vaginal atrophy related to aromatase inhibitors: a phase I/II study. Oncologist 16:424–431
62. Pfaus JG (2009) Pathways of sexual desire. J Sex Med 6:1506–1533
63. Arnow BA, Millheiser L, Garrett A, Lake Polan M, Glover GH, Hill KR et al (2009) Women with hypoactive sexual desire disorder compared to normal females: a functional magnetic resonance imaging study. Neuroscience 158:484–502
64. Stahl SM, Sommer B, Allers KA (2011) Multifunctional pharmacology of flibanserin: possible mechanism of therapeutic action in hypoactive sexual desire disorder. J Sex Med 8:15–27
65. Simon JA, Kingsberg SA, Shumel B, Hanes V, Garcia M Jr, Sand M (2013) Efficacy and safety of flibanserin in postmenopausal women with hypoactive sexual desire disorder: results of the SNOWDROP trial. Menopause 21:633–640
66. Derogatis LR, Komer L, Katz M, Moreau M, Kimura T, Garcia M Jr et al (2012) Treatment of hypoactive sexual desire disorder in premenopausal women: efficacy of flibanserin in the VIOLET study. J Sex Med 9:1074–1085
67. Thorp J, Simon J, Dattani D, Taylor L, Kimura T, Garcia M Jr et al (2012) Treatment of hypoactive sexual desire disorder in premenopausal women: efficacy of flibanserin in the DAISY study. J Sex Med 9:793–804
68. Katz M, DeRogatis LR, Ackerman R, Hedges P, Lesko L, Garcia M Jr et al (2013) Efficacy of flibanserin in women with hypoactive sexual desire disorder: results from the BEGONIA trial. J Sex Med 10:1807–1815
69. Joffe HV, Chang C, Sewell C, Easley O, Nguyen C, Dunn S et al (2016) fda approval of flibanserin-treating hypoactive sexual desire disorder. N Engl J Med 374:101–104
70. Molinoff PB, Shadiack AM, Earle D, Diamond LE, Quon CY (2003) PT-141: a melanocortin agonist for the treatment of sexual dysfunction. Ann NY Acad Sci 994:96–102

71. Diamond LE, Earle DC, Heiman JR, Rosen RC, Perelman MA, Harning R (2006) An effect on the subjective sexual response in premenopausal women with sexual arousal disorder by bremelanotide (PT-141), a melanocortin receptor agonist. J Sex Med 3:628–638
72. Clayton AH, Althof SE, Kingsberg S, DeRogatis LR, Kroll R, Goldstein I et al (2016) Bremelanotide for female sexual dysfunctions in premenopausal women: a randomized, placebo-controlled dose-finding trial. Womens Health (Lond) 12:325–337
73. Abstracts of the ACOG (American College of Obstetricians and Gynecologists) (2008) 56th annual clinical meeting. May 3–7, 2008. New Orleans, Louisiana, USA. Obstet Gynecol 111:1S–113S
74. Bremelanotide Meets Co-Primary Endpoints in Palatin's Phase 3 Trials for Hypoactive Sexual Desire Disorder. Available at: http://www.prnewswire.com/news-releases/bremelanotide-meets-co-primary-endpoints-in-palatins-phase-3-trials-for-hypoactive-sexual-desire-disorder-300355401.html [cited 2017 01/29/2017]

Patient References (Books)

75. Streicher L Sex Rx: hormones, health and your best sex ever
76. Goldstein A, Pukall C, Goldstein I (2011) When sex hurts: a woman's guide to banishing sexual pain. Perseus Books
77. Pendergast S (2016) Pelvic pain explained. Rowman & Littlefield Publishers
78. American Association of Sex Educators, Counselors, and Therapists (AASECT). www.aasect.org to find a therapist trained in couple's therapy and sexual function
79. North American Menopause Society. www.menopause.org
80. American Congress of Obstetricians and Gynecologists Guide to Midlife Health: www.pause.acog.org
81. International Pelvic Pain Society. www.pelvicpain.org
82. Vaginismus: Helping Women Overcome Sexual Pain. www.vaginismus.com

CPSIA information can be obtained
at www.ICGtesting.com
Printed in the USA
LVHW082137060619
620471LV00004B/362/P